Overcoming Dyslexia

Overcoming Dyslexia

IN CHILDREN, ADOLESCENTS, AND ADULTS

DALE R. JORDAN

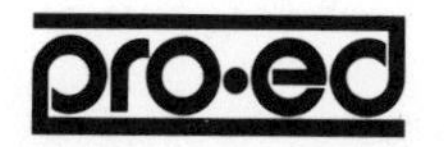

8700 Shoal Creek Boulevard
Austin, Texas 78758

Printed in the United States of America

Published by arrangement with Modern Education Corporation

Library of Congress Cataloging-in-Publication Data

Jordan, Dale R.
Overcoming dyslexia.

Bibliography: p.
Includes index.
1. Dyslexia—Popular works. I. Title. [DNLM: Dyslexia—therapy. WM 475 J82o]
RC394.W6J67 1989 616.85'53 89-3958
ISBN 0-89079-204-6

pro·ed

8700 Shoal Creek Boulevard
Austin, Texas 78758

10 9 8 7 6 5 4 3 2 1 89 90 91 92 93

Contents

Preface

> "Every man has a train of thought on which he rides when he is alone. The dignity and nobility of his life, as well as his happiness, depend upon the direction in which that train is going, the baggage it carries, and the scenery through which it travels."
>
> *Joseph Fort Newton*

I began teaching struggling learners in Lincoln Elementary School 30 years ago. As a newly certified classroom teacher, I had no idea about learning disabilities. Like most mainstream classroom teachers then and now, I watched helplessly as certain youngsters struggled so hard to read, spell, write, do assignments, and earn praise through their work. But no matter how hard they tried, they never could achieve grade level competency. Through the past three decades, I have kept in touch with many of my first students. I have watched them become adults, and now I am involved with their children. This two-generation experience has let me see the kind of baggage these strugglers tend to carry into their adult lives, and it is not always good. The scenery through which their adult "train" travels is often filled with failure and heartache. Several of my early students are serving prison sentences. Many have gone through divorce. I have lost count of how many became addicted to drugs and alcohol. I just did not know what to do for them back in the 1950s. And all too few classroom teachers of the 1980s know much more now than my generation did three decades ago.

During the 1960s an explosion of new knowledge began to take place in our understanding of specific learning disability. Such notable pioneers as Beth Slingerland, Samuel Kirk, Marianne Frostig, and Sam Clements began to identify specific patterns of learning dysfunction that pointed the way to better education for young strugglers. At the same time, medical science began to delve into how brain functions affect academic learning, following the lead of such early researchers as Samuel Orton. By 1988 an incredible wealth of new knowledge was available about brain-based dysfunctions, especially about dyslexia. As we near the end of the 20th century, we have at hand knowledge and technology no one dreamed of when I was a young teacher 30 years ago.

In November 1985 the Menninger Foundation in Topeka, Kansas, sponsored a forum that brought together a remarkable cross section of professionals who deal with learning disabilities. Drake Duane, a neurologist with the Mayo Clinic School of Medicine, made a truly startling statement when he said: "Dyslexia is now the most thoroughly researched of all the various learning disabilities" (Duane 1979, 1985). A little time spent in library research proves his statement true. For example, in 1982 an ambitious book was published entitled *Dyslexia: An Annotated Bibliography*, by Martha M. Evans. Evans had reviewed all of the published information she could find regarding dyslexia. She culled out material that did not seem carefully enough written to be beneficial. This left her with more than 2,500 articles and publications about the problem of dyslexia. Since 1982 hundreds of additional articles and books have been published on this topic.

During the 1980s several internationally renowned "giants" in research of dyslexia have appeared. Those who attend symposia sponsored by The Orton Dyslexia Society and the Association for Children and Adults with Learning Disability (ACLD) are familiar with the exciting research reported by Albert Galaburda of Harvard Medical School, Martha Denckla of Johns Hopkins School of Medicine, Bruce McEwen of the Rockefeller University School of Medicine, Drake Duane of the Mayo Foundation, Sondra Jernigan from the Menninger Foundation, Veronika Grimm from the Weizmann Institute of Science in Israel, the late Norman Geschwind of Harvard Medical School, William Deering and Jane Flynn from LaCrosse (Wisconsin) Lutheran Hospital, Antonio R. Damasio of the University of Iowa College of Medicine, and many more. These leaders in research have shown us the tip of the iceberg regarding the organic causes of dyslexia and related learning or behavioral problems. It is truly astonishing how much knowledge is emerging about struggling learners, especially the dyslexic population.

This book is not intended to be a scientific treatise about dyslexia. There are many excellent publications that present that kind of clinical data. The purpose of *Overcoming Dyslexia in Children, Adolescents, and Adults* is to translate the mysteries of specialized clinical data into "everyday language" for parents, students, classroom teachers, tutors, and anyone else who needs more practical knowledge of this critical issue. The references at the end of this book will direct you to more technical writing, if that is what you need or prefer. This book is an attempt to translate research knowledge into a simple, practical form. To paraphrase ancient mythology, my goal is to bring fire down from Olympus for the benefit of those who do not have the time or the background to translate research language for themselves.

1

The Nature of Dyslexia

The decade of the 1970s in American education started with a bombshell that shattered many assumptions. The Nixon administration issued an in-depth study of the level of literacy in the adult population of the United States at the close of the 1960s. An astonishing fact was reported: Approximately 25 million men and women between the ages of 18 and 55 were illiterate. This segment of the labor market could not read a restaurant menu, follow a road map successfully, interpret street signs, fill out job application forms without help, apply for a Social Security card on their own, fill out papers for government assistance, read a newspaper, or help their children with homework assignments. As this news about the presence of illiteracy in our culture made its impact, other studies revealed that as many as one-third of all public school students dropped out before finishing high school. On looking back over school records, several states discovered that since before World War II, public high schools had been losing one-third of their students before graduation. During the 1970s more than 70 literacy studies were done with the population of adjudicated delinquents and adult males serving prison sentences. It was discovered that three out of four adjudicated or incarcerated males could not read, write, or spell above third-grade level. Not only was our national labor market teeming with illiterate adults, but our prison systems were also crowded by those who could not function on their own with tasks requiring fourth grade or higher literacy skills.

An obvious question was still being debated during the 1988 presidential campaign: How could the most productive nation on earth produce such an astonishing number of educational failures? How could we possibly have failed to educate such vast numbers of men and women?

No reasonable person would infer that dyslexia is the sole cause for this much illiteracy in our culture. Dyslexia is only one of several forms of specific learning disability. As Martha Denckla (1985) has pointed out, illiterate persons may have several overlapping problems that keep them from mastering literacy skills. Some illiterates are dyslexic, although as late as 1988 no one knew how many dysfunctional adults might be dyslexic. Residual Attention Deficit Disorder is often a factor in low literacy skills, but we do not know how many adults are learning disabled by attention deficit problems. As Geiger and Lettvin (1987) have shown, poor central vision is often an inhibiting factor in learning to read and write. We do not know how many persons in our culture have been academically disabled by mental illness. Obviously, social and economic deprivation can be major factors in illiteracy. Clearly, there is no single reason why 25 million of our adult citizens are illiterate.

Definitions and Descriptions

I began my work with struggling learners more than 30 years ago before American education included the concepts of learning disability and dyslexia. For the past three decades I have observed and participated in the effort to define language dysfunction in our culture. It has not been easy for professional groups to reach consensus on the definition of dyslexia or specific learning disability. Progress has been made toward a common definition of these problems, but a survey of recent professional literature still shows wide differences of opinion among physicians, psychologists, psychiatrists, educators, and psychometrists as to what dyslexia is and how it should be defined. Those who are interested in research are often dissatisfied by the rather general definitions offered by educators. Teachers are often frustrated by technical definitions developed by researchers. As Evans (1982) demonstrated in her review of 2,500 studies of dyslexia, more than 200 definitions of this problem were generated by professionals before 1982. Many newer definitions have been offered during the 1980s by such groups as The Orton Dyslexia Society, Association for Children and Adults with Learning Disability (ACLD), National Joint Committee for Learning Disabilities (NJCLD), and Council for Learning Disabilities (CLD).

For example, Critchley (1970) defined dyslexia as follows:

> A disorder manifested by difficulty in learning to read despite conventional instruction, adequate intelligence, and socio-cultural opportunity. It is dependent upon fundamental cognitive disabilities which are frequently of constitutional origin. (p. 11)

This definition was roundly criticized by such researchers as Inouye and Sorenson (1985), who gave five reasons why this kind of simplification is inadequate. In sharp contrast to Critchley's simplicity is the definition of dyslexia developed by the International Reading Association (Harris & Hodges, 1981):

> Dyslexia
> 1. n. A medical term for incomplete alexia; partial but severe, inability to read; historically (but less common in current use), word blindness. Note: Dyslexia in this sense applies to persons who ordinarily have adequate vision, hearing, intelligence, and general language functioning. Dyslexia is a rare but definable and diagnosable form of primary reading retardation with some form of central nervous system dysfunction. It is not attributable to environmental causes or other handicapping conditions.
>
> 2. n. A severe reading disability of unexpected origin.
>
> 3. n. A popular term for any difficulty in reading of any intensity and from any cause(s). Note: Dyslexia in this sense is a term which describes a symptom, not a disease. (p. 95)

Hynd and Cohen (1983) regard this kind of definition of dyslexia as "exemplary." Other equally qualified researchers do not (Gray & Kavanagh, 1985). Public agencies which must deal with large numbers of struggling learners and poor readers often do not accept any definition or explanation of dyslexia. Parents who move to different areas of the United States are often frustrated by lack of agreement among educators regarding the issue of dyslexia. For example, in 1985 the 69th Texas Legislature adopted House Bills 157 and 2168, which required public schools to screen all students for dyslexia. The following definition of dyslexia is now the official educational point of reference for the State of Texas:

> A disorder of constitutional origin manifested by difficulty in learning to read, write or spell, despite conventional instruction, adequate intelligence, and socio-cultural opportunity. (Orton Dyslexia Society, 1988, p. 2)

Meanwhile, north of the Red River from Texas, the states of Oklahoma and Kansas do not recognize dyslexia as a learning disability.

If a Texas child is diagnosed as being dyslexic according to Texas definition, he or she would be placed in a special educational program designed to meet that specific need. If that child should move to Oklahoma or Kansas, the Texas designation would not be recognized as a reason for special education placement. Obviously, there is a long way to go before the issue of dyslexia is universally defined and recognized among professionals in the United States.

In spite of these differences of opinion, it is possible to describe learning disability. In American culture, learning disability is a cluster of factors that keeps an intelligent child from learning how to do school work successfully. As such students move upward through the grades, they do not develop fluent skills in reading from printed materials. It is impossible for these students to do typical reading assignments expected by adults. They cannot write effectively. Penmanship is poor. Fine motor coordination never becomes smooth in controlling the pencil or pen. Sentence structure is ragged and incomplete. These students usually have trouble copying accurately from the chalkboard or from a book. They seldom do well with basic arithmetic. These students must count fingers to add, subtract, multiply, or divide. They usually need to whisper over and over while their fingers touch or handle the work page. Rate of work is usually very slow. These students become intensely frustrated if adults try to make them work faster. Vision problems are seen as their eyes become overly tired after a few minutes of close work. The ability to see details clearly at desk-top level deteriorates. Within a few minutes these students must look away, rub their eyes, or start using a marker to keep their place on the page. Attention span is often very short, causing these students to dart off on rabbit trails instead of keeping the attention focused fully on the task. These students usually listen poorly. They cannot keep up with a flow of oral information. They usually cannot follow directions that involve memory for left and right. They usually become confused with the concepts of north, south, east, and west. They are often much less mature than their age-mates, which creates conflict with peers and adults. These struggling students do very poorly on tests, especially when time is limited. They are frequently misdiagnosed as being mentally retarded or emotionally disturbed because they cannot give coherent standard responses on diagnostic tests. This "special population" exists in virtually every classroom and community in the United States. Yet they have not been adequately identified or treated effectively by our system of education. It is easy to describe learning disability. Creating an acceptable definition is another matter.

Forms of Learning Disability

We now recognize several forms of learning disability. It would be more accurate to say that we see specific variations of the same struggle to acquire an education. Some professionals see what is generally called "minimal brain dysfunction," usually designated as MBD. This refers to a cluster of behaviors including hyperactivity, very poor organization ability, spotty and unpredictable ability to master basic academic skills, short attention span, and numerous "soft neurological signs" that include poor fine motor coordination, awkward gross motor coordination, and poor ability of the eyes to team together for accurate focusing and refocusing. MBD is often medicated to reduce hyperactivity and increase attention span. Those who follow this point of view tend to regard MBD children as being emotionally unstable and hard to educate. The designation minimal brain dysfunction is often not very helpful, other than to give a name to a certain cluster of behavior problems.

Attention Deficit Disorder

In 1980 the American Psychiatric Association published the third edition of its Diagnostic and Statistical Manual (DMS III) (American Psychiatric Association, 1980). A new category of learning disability emerged. DSM III introduced the concept of Attention Deficit Disorder in three subcategories: (1) Attention Deficit Disorder with Hyperactivity; (2) Attention Deficit Disorder without Hyperactivity; and (3) Attention Deficit Disorder, Residual Type. Professionals began referring to ADD or ADD Syndrome. Later this clear, easily understood diagnostic guideline was changed by a revision called DSM III-R (American Psychiatric Association, 1987). As Kutchins and Kirk (1988) have described, DSM III-R has created a storm of controversy within the diagnostic arena. According to the changes of DSM III-R, the three earlier categories of Attention Deficit Disorder were lumped together as a single syndrome: Attention Deficit/Hyperactive Disorder (ADHD). The 1987 revision of APA guidelines eliminated two important categories of Attention Deficit Disorder (without Hyperactivity and Residual Type). To qualify for the new ADHD diagnosis, a child or adult must show 8 out of 14 behavior patterns. Oddly, only 5 of the 14 criteria refer to hyperactivity. DSM III-R leaves the diagnostician in the difficult position of reporting certain children or adults as "nonhyperactive/hyperactive." The original subcategories of Attention Deficit Disorder without Hyperactivity and Residual Type are now buried inside new terminology, yet they still exist within the diagnostic criteria of DSM III-R.

In spite of the 1987 changes in diagnostic nomenclature, we still see three forms of Attention Deficit Disorder, as DSM III (1980) correctly described. Attention Deficit Disorder refers to the student who cannot keep attention focused on an academic task. No matter how hard the student tries, his or her attention darts or drifts away to another issue instead of staying on the assigned task. This student may or may not be hyperactive. A common mistake is made by diagnosticians who assume that ADD Syndrome always includes hyperactivity. As Hagerman (1983) and Jordan (1988) have described, many of the attention drifters are not hyperactive but are often passive and withdrawn in the classroom. ADD Syndrome is marked by certain definite behavior patterns: short attention span; cluttered impressions of new information; continual distraction by what is going on nearby; frequent conflict with others; chronic messiness and cluttered space; inability to remember details or carry out responsibilities; need for constant supervision; extremely poor listening comprehension; often good reading ability for short periods of time; usually good phonics skills, but inability to apply that knowledge in a meaningful way. The ADD Syndrome student, whether hyperactive or passive, appears irresponsible, scatter-brained, unreliable, lazy, and unproductive. Most students with this pattern are misfits with immature social skills. If they do not outgrow these patterns during adolescence, they become terribly frustrated, unsuccessful adults who cannot keep a job, hold a marriage together, be good parents, or contribute to society in a productive way. Attention Deficit Disorder is found in most classrooms and communities. The irony is that few definitions of learning disability include this frequently seen problem. Few Attention Deficit Disorder students are included in special programs for learning disabled youngsters.

Dyslexia

There is a specific form of learning disability that, according to Duane (1985), has become the most thoroughly researched problem of all. This is dyslexia. Several pioneers in the field of neurological research have documented the organic causes of this specific learning disability more carefully than any other educational problem. In the early 1920s Samuel Orton began to see specific patterns in brain-damaged adults who at one time could read, spell, and write adequately. After sustaining brain injury, they reversed letters, read words backwards, forgot how to spell, and stumbled over basic math computation. Dr. Orton's pioneering research shortly after World War I blazed the trail for understanding this mysterious problem that caused reading failure, spelling disability, handwriting difficulty, and arithmetic struggle. Dr. Orton demonstrated that certain areas of the left brain are involved in these academic skills. He showed us that when certain left brain areas are damaged, these specific academic skills are retarded or blocked. Today the Orton Society carries on the research started half a century ago by this insightful neurologist.

In the late 1970s a remarkable neurologist at Harvard Medical School became deeply interested in the controversial issue of dyslexia. The late Dr. Norman Geschwind started a series of research projects designed to see whether dyslexia in fact exists, or whether it is just one of those myths that emerge from time to time. He enlisted the help of several talented colleagues, including Albert Galaburda, Antonio Damasio, and Drake Duane. Galaburda has performed a series of brain autopsies using the brains of dyslexic men. His studies have given us proof that certain neuronal structures are different in the brains of dyslexics (Galaburda, 1983). Specific areas of the left brain where language concepts, printed symbols, and math information are processed do not develop normally. In the dyslexic brain, there are structural differences in those areas that govern the development of literacy skills.

As these facts of dyslexic brain differences have become known, a variety of diagnostic tools have been developed to identify dyslexia according to brain wave patterns and the way specific areas of the brain respond to stimulus. Sondra Jernigan at the Menninger Foundation in Topeka, Kansas, has pioneered evoked potential EEG measurements to identify certain forms of primary dyslexia. William Deering and Jane Flynn at LaCrosse Lutheran Hospital in LaCrosse, Wisconsin, have developed ways to see dyslexia in the theta band of an EEG evaluation. Other researchers are developing techniques through CAT, PET, MRI, and other kinds of brain wave evaluation to pinpoint the neurological signatures of dyslexia in the brain. Biochemical research at centers such as the Weizmann Institute of Science in Israel, under the direction of Veronika Grimm, is showing us that body chemistry is also an important factor when dyslexia exists. Geschwind's studies yielded a profile of the families of dyslexics. In a majority of cases there is a much higher than normal incidence of left-handedness within the genetic family structure. Relatives of dyslexics tend to become gray-haired or white-haired at early ages. Allergies are prevalent within dyslexic families, as is the tendency for gastrointestinal problems and digestive sensitivity. Dyslexic families have a higher than normal level of autoimmune disorders in which the body tends to attack itself. We now know that dyslexia is tied to physical patterns within the person's brain as well as to the body chemistry and genetic traits of certain families. It is not caused by poor teaching, poor parenting, or lack of cultural opportunity. Dyslexia is found in all human cultures. It has no ethnic or economic preference. It is noticed in all cultures where literacy skills are important.

Dyslexia is a complex condition. Popular opinion holds that dyslexic persons reverse the letter *b* and *d* and read words backwards (*saw* for *was*). This overly simple view says that if a student does not reverse letters or words, then he or she is not dyslexic. That kind of oversimplification is dangerously misleading. Like any other human condition, there is nothing simple about dyslexia. It is seen in a variety of ways on many levels of severity. Some dyslexics do reverse letters, numbers, and words. Many do not. Being dyslexic is much more complex than getting a few symbols backwards.

At this point it would be helpful to give my own definition of dyslexia. As has already been pointed out, there is no universally accepted definition of this condition. Each group with a vested interest in this problem will arrive at its own definition. In her book *Dyslexia: An Annotated Bibliography,* Martha Evans (1982) reviewed more than 200 definitions of dyslexia, most of them in agreement concerning the basic characteristics of the syndrome, but each definition differing from the others according to each author's perception of the problem. Earlier in this chapter we saw three sample definitions of dyslexia reflecting different points of view. Based upon my own 30 years of one-to-one experience with the dyslexic population, I have developed the following definition:

> Dyslexia is the inability of an intelligent person to become fluent in the basic skills of reading, spelling, and handwriting in spite of prolonged teaching and tutoring. Math computation may also remain at the level of struggle. Dyslexia means that the person will always struggle to some degree reading printed passages, writing with a pen or pencil, spelling accurately from memory, and developing sentences and paragraphs with correct grammar and punctuation. Dyslexia may also include difficulty telling information orally as well as listening to oral information accurately. No matter how hard the person tries, certain types of errors continue to appear in reading, writing, and spelling. Dyslexia is a brain-based dysfunction that is often genetic. It tends to run in families. Through certain kinds of remedial training, dyslexic patterns can be partly overcome or reduced, but dyslexia cannot be completely eliminated. It is a lifelong, brain-based condition that most dyslexics can learn to compensate for successfully.

Levels of Dyslexia

It is important that a certain point of view be maintained as we think of dyslexia. No two dyslexic persons display exactly the same patterns, and not all dyslexic persons show the same level of severity. The cluster of dyslexic patterns must be seen along a continuum from mild to severe. Many dyslexics show only mild or moderate problems, while others are severely disabled. Dyslexia should be seen along the following continuum:

0	1	2	3	4	5	6	7	8	9	10
none		mild				moderate			severe	

Most adults would show a few dyslexic-like "blips" in their literacy and math skills. In one sense, it would be correct to say that each of us is dyslexic at Level 1 or Level 2. Few persons have perfect literacy skills without some area of deficit. That poses no problem so long as those specific problems do not create costly mistakes on the job. Adults typically choose professions or occupations that permit them to bypass whatever minor deficits exist in spelling, rapid recall of details, rapid math processing, and so forth.

Dyslexia becomes an educational problem when it begins to interfere with classroom performance and academic success. Moderate dyslexia at Level 4 or Level 5 would mean continual mistakes in spelling, punctuation, and capital letters; grammar errors; mistakes in reading comprehension; and many small errors in math computation. A moderately dyslexic student would struggle with every written assignment, but he or she could finally do good work by trying hard enough and rewriting papers two or three times. With enough effort, Level 4 and Level 5 dyslexics can make top grades and be listed on the honor roll, but they must maintain a high level of self-discipline to do so.

When dyslexia is at Level 6 or Level 7, a major struggle is seen in all areas of academic performance. Spelling is always faulty, textbook reading is slow and difficult, much more time than usual is required to finish homework assignments, and a high level of personal frustration is experienced. Level 6 and Level 7 dyslexics reach burnout before they can finish their assignments. They must continually deal with a sense of failure and discouragement. Occasionally they earn top grades, but they usually show only average or below average performance on report cards. It is seldom possible for a Level 6 or Level 7 dyslexic student to make the school's honor roll or to win praise for academic achievement. It is possible for a dyslexic student at this level to finish a college degree, but it requires great effort and courage to do so.

When dyslexia exists at the severe level (Level 8 or Level 9), academic achievement is often impossible unless teachers modify the curriculum for those students. Occasionally we find a Level 10 student where the disability is so severe that academic learning is impossible. That condition is referred to as *alexia*. A dyslexic student at Level 8 or Level 9 will be several years below grade level in skill achievement. That student cannot spell above a primitive level. Reading is a massive struggle. Handwriting is poor and messy. It usually requires two to three times longer than normal for a Level 8 or Level 9 dyslexic to finish typical assignments, and he or she must have continual help to do so. It is virtually impossible for these students to attain independent study skills. They must have continual tutoring and coaching to prepare for tests, do assignments, master new information, and fill in gaps in their skills and knowledge. If these students are taught to do their writing through a word processor, they can bypass enough dyslexic problems to turn out good work through the keyboard. With a hand calculator they can do good math. But it is impossible for them to function academically through the traditional mode of silent reading, producing handwritten papers, and turning out large quantities of work day after day. Level 8 and Level 9 dyslexics suffer continually from the self-image that they are "dumb." They almost never win praise for their academic work. They have no good stories to tell about classroom achievement. Unless they excel in athletics or art, these students languish through their school years with intense feelings of failure and low self-worth.

Forms of Dyslexia

Most of the professional controversy about dyslexia is caused by misunderstanding as to which form of dyslexia one is referring. There are three general forms of this learning disability. It is of critical importance that different forms of dyslexia are recognized. If only one form is acknowledged, then it becomes impossible for professionals to discuss the issue effectively.

Trauma Induced Dyslexia

One form of dyslexia is directly related to brain damage. Certain areas of the brain are irreversibly damaged through experiences that destroy brain tissue, such as overdose of drugs; loss of oxygen over a period of time; stroke; debilitating disease such as Alzheimer's, which produces senility; industrial or automobile accidents; athletic accidents; and neurological damage at birth. As Dr. Orton demonstrated many years ago, these kinds of trauma to the brain tissues can produce a dyslexic syndrome (reversal of symbols, loss of phonics, inability to keep details in sequence, inability to connect sounds to letters, loss of reading comprehension, inability to spell). This definition of dyslexia applies only to a small segment of our population (less than 1%). If this brain-damage model of dyslexia is the only one considered, then there is no explanation for the millions of other dyslexics who exist within the population but who show no signs of brain damage. A great deal of confusion is generated when the brain-damage model of dyslexia is the only point of reference. This definition was never intended to address the problems faced by parents and classroom teachers in dealing with dyslexic problems among students.

Primary Dyslexia

A second form of dyslexia runs in families. We now know that it is carried by Chromosome 15 in the genetic chain, and it appears approximately nine times more often in men than in women. From 3% to 5% of the general population have primary dyslexia. We are deeply indebted to Norman Geschwind (1979, 1983, 1984, 1985) and Albert Galaburda (1983) of Harvard Medical School for their postmortem studies of several dyslexic brains. They found specific areas of the left brain (within the left cerebral cortex) that are different from those same areas in nondyslexic brains. The term *primary dyslexia* refers to deep-seated trouble with reading comprehension, sounding out words, spelling, writing legibly, learning to do math from memory, pronouncing words without tongue twisting, and creating written material with correct grammar, punctuation, and sentence structure. This form of dyslexia does not improve with age or physical maturity. At age 40 most primary dyslexics still struggle to read below fourth-grade level, and spelling is almost impossible to achieve. This form of dyslexia is seen in other blood relatives, usually males. It can skip a generation if passed along by the mother. A grandfather and his male relatives can be dyslexic but his daughter not show significant signs. Her son (the third generation) can be severely dyslexic and pass the pattern on down the family line. Relatives of primary dyslexics show much higher levels of allergies than normal, and they have more digestive problems (duodenal ulcers, colitis, Crohn's Disease). Relatives of primary dyslexics tend to turn gray or white-haired at early ages, and a high percentage of those relatives are left-handed.

Secondary Dyslexia

The third form of dyslexia has two names: secondary dyslexia or developmental dyslexia. This form of dyslexia may also run in families, although it can appear when no other relatives show the symptoms. Secondary dyslexia is seen in 12% to 15% of the general population. Research by Grimm (1986) at the Weizmann Institute of Science in Israel indicates that this form of dyslexia is caused early in the development of the fetus. Toward the end of the first trimester of fetal development, the tiny cells that later become the genitals produce a surge of male hormone (testosterone). This occurs long before the baby is physically either male or female. At this stage of fetal development, the brain still has not taken shape. Groups of cells that later become the right brain and left brain hemispheres are migrating upward toward the developing head of the fetus. The surge of testosterone temporarily stops development of the left brain cells, while the right brain cells continue to develop on schedule. This produces an imbalance in brain development. Later the left brain hemisphere catches up. In fact, the left brain hemisphere of the dyslexic person is the same size as the right brain hemisphere. In nondyslexic brains, the right brain hemisphere is somewhat larger. This surge of male hormone near the end of the first trimester of fetal development sets the stage for the differences seen later when brains of dyslexic students are studied.

Secondary dyslexia or developmental dyslexia is caused by late development of the language processing centers of the left brain hemisphere. In this form of dyslexia, the struggle to learn gradually decreases as the child goes through puberty. The hormones that bring about body changes during puberty finish "filling in" the language centers of the left brain of dyslexic students. As this late maturity of brain tissue takes place, the level of dyslexia drops. Most secondary dyslexics begin to break through their learning problems about age 12 as hormone production gets under way. By age 14 they are usually much better able to handle school learning. By age 16 their academic skills are noticeably better, with math, reading comprehension, and language skills showing much improvement. During their early twenties these students show remarkable gains in learning ability, compared with their struggle during elementary school and middle school years. Most secondary dyslexics are able to do well in college if self-esteem has not been too badly damaged during their early struggles in school.

As has been pointed out earlier, dyslexia is seen as a continuum, not as a single level of difficulty. The syndrome ranges widely in complexity from student to student. On the scale of 0 to 10, primary dyslexics are usually at the severe level (8 or 9), meaning that some ability to master basic literacy skills exists. Secondary dyslexics usually fall in the moderate range (4 through 7). If a secondary dyslexic student is identified at Level 7 during the elementary school years, he or she may have improved to Level 5 by age 16. He or she may show further improvement by age 20 or 21. Developmental dyslexia (secondary dyslexia) usually involves less learning difficulty as the central nervous system finishes maturing during adolescence. It is not unusual to see a student who is at Level 7 at age 10 be down to Level 4 by age 20. As the severity of the syndrome decreases during puberty, academic performance rises if appropriate remedial training is provided.

Continual controversy exists when it comes to saying how many dyslexic persons there are in our society. Estimates range from very few to as many as 20% of the population. My own estimate is that from 12% to 15% of the population shows significant signs of dyslexic spelling, writing, reading, and math struggle (Jordan, 1977, 1988b). This does not mean that 12 or 15 people out of every 100 are clinically dyslexic. As Denckla (1985) has described, those of us who work closely with the learning disabled population see much overlapping of problems. It is rare to find a struggling student who manifests only one specific form of disability. This is well illustrated by Alston and Taylor (1987) as they show handwriting samples of children who have been diagnosed as having spina bifida, petit mal epilepsy, spastic quadriplegia, ataxia, cerebellar lesion, Duchenne muscular dystrophy, and osteogenesis imperfecta. In each of their illustrations, difficulty with handwriting (dysgraphia) is seen, along with poor spelling that would fit the patterns of dyslexic spellers. The difficulty in assigning percentage figures to the prevalence of any form of learning disability is not recognizing overlapping conditions. I have seldom seen a dyslexic student who was brain injured according to EEG or CAT scan investigation. However, I have worked with many brain-injured persons who had dyslexic-like literacy problems. A survey of the literature of the past 15 years finds most writers agreeing with the estimate that approximately 15% of our population manifest dyslexic patterns in basic literacy skill mastery.

Dyslexic children do not automatically master language symbols, and they do not automatically perceive left to right and top to bottom. Some dyslexics cannot handle the processes involved in translating spoken language into written symbols, often referred to as "encoding." Such children cannot change what they hear into an accurate written code. Other dyslexics have difficulty translating printed symbols into meaning. They are unable to "decode" what they see in printed form. Still others cannot express themselves in writing because they cannot remember how to make specific letters correctly. These students cannot control the direction of written symbols, which makes very poor handwriting. These forms of learning disability are complicated by the tendency to interpret symbols backwards, upside down, and in scrambled sequence.

The major difficulty in the classroom, however, is that few students are handicapped by only one form of dyslexia. Two or more kinds of this perceptual loss usually exist in dyslexic students. These clusters of perceptual handicaps make it all the more difficult for the disability to be corrected. In fact, severe cases of dyslexia (Level 8 or Level 9) require special clinical treatment, which a regular classroom cannot possibly provide. It is essential that teachers be able to screen their pupils in order to make the necessary referrals for those who need specialized help. Moderately dyslexic students (Level 4 through Level 7) can be taught successfully within the mainstream classroom structure, if teachers make certain adjustments in assignments and learning procedures.

Visual Dyslexia. The most obvious form of dyslexic handicap is that of visual dyslexia. This is basically the inability to interpret printed language symbols. The visual dyslexic student struggles to change printed messages into inner speech. He or she often cannot connect what is seen on the page to what is said in conversation. Visual dyslexia is not caused by poor vision. Students with severe visual impairment are not dyslexic because of poor eyesight. Visual dyslexia is not a matter of seeing poorly; it is a matter of the brain not interpreting accurately what is seen.

Poor central vision. Since the days when Dr. Orton did his pioneering studies of dyslexics, those of us who have worked with this special population have seen a puzzling vision tendency that is seldom identified during typical vision examinations (Greenstein, 1976; Leisman, 1976; Rayner, 1983). Tutors and remedial teachers have long contended that dyslexics have a different way of seeing as they read. Yet this point of view has been disputed by ophthalmologists and many optometrists because the standard techniques used in vision examination do not identify this irregular visual pattern. Two enterprising researchers at the Massachusetts Institute of Technology have verified the fact that most dyslexics do indeed see differently when they try to read. In most instances, this different way of seeing is a critical block in developing reading skills. Geiger and Lettvin (1987) have shown that most dyslexics have poor foveal (central) vision to decode the printed page. The foveal region of each eye gathers incoming visual information, then transmits it to the visual cortex at the back of the head where the brain interprets what we see. In normal reading, the peripheral images (what the eyes see at the edge of the visual field) are ignored by the brain. The visual cortex in normal readers tunes out or ignores the periphery and concentrates on what is seen by the central (foveal) vision. In many dyslexics, the eyes do not see printed details straight ahead. Instead, the eyes of most dyslexics see at an angle, or off center. If the student is to see a printed word clearly, he or she must actually focus at an angle away from the word but not directly at the word.

Geiger and Lettvin (1987) have documented this peripheral vision of dyslexic students. They have shown that most dyslexics cannot see to read in a normal way. This is why most dyslexic students need to mark as they read. By running a finger or pencil beneath the line, by framing words with two fingers, or by reading with a card that has a slot cut out, dyslexics can handle the visual work of reading. If they must decode a page without this kind of compensation, they cannot see printed details clearly. This new evidence helps to explain why many dyslexics resist trying to read. They cannot see words on the page without learning to focus from an angle along with developing a marking system to guide their eyes along the lines of print.

Reversing and scrambling details. Most visual dyslexics also see certain letters backwards or upside down. Reading whole words in sentences is a jumbled process for such a student. Not only do dyslexic students perceive individual letters incorrectly, but they also see parts of words backwards. When these dyslexic idiosyncrasies are at work during reading, students have a disorganized, meaningless, and usually frustrating experience. Consequently, they do everything possible to avoid reading. For example, Paul, who is handicapped by visual dyslexia, is asked to read the following paragraph silently:

> Down the cold, dark stairs crept the man in the black coat. Closer he came, closer and closer. Asleep in their blankets, Dan and Pete were unaware of their danger.

Because of reversals, sequence scrambling, and failure to pick up details, this is Paul's perception of the paragraph the first time he reads it:

> Now the could, back stars keep the man in the dalk coat. Colser he come, colser and colser sheeping the dantes anD and deer wore nuraw for the bang.

In order to do this reading, Paul touches the words with his finger and whispers each word to himself. The teacher, who is unaware of the nature of Paul's reading disability, has made an issue of marking and whispering. She snaps her fingers and says "Shhhhhh!" when he whispers as he reads. The teacher does not realize that, by cutting off Paul's speaking-listening channels, she has made it impossible for him to check his visual impressions against what he hears. The result is complete nonsense for Paul, and he flunks still another comprehension quiz because of silent reading. Had he been allowed to whisper the words, thus checking them against his listening vocabulary, he could have worked out the meaning of the passage at his usual slow pace.

Because of this sort of scrambled perception, visual dyslexics are forced to work very slowly. This slowness is a factor usually misunderstood by teachers and parents. If the typical student in Paul's class can digest the above passage in 3 minutes, it may take him as long as 15 minutes. The demands for speed in reading and writing are being increased by the pressures of the modern curriculum, but visual dyslexics cannot work rapidly. When they are placed with impatient instructors or tutors who do not understand their problems, students like Paul have no way of coping with their assigned reading tasks.

Because visual dyslexics have such a constant problem handling information in sequence, they usually have trouble with basic arithmetic. Learning to add, subtract, multiply, and divide involves frequent changes in direction that are opposite from the left-to-right, top-to-bottom orientation stressed in reading and writing. To add, Paul must start at the right side of the problem and work downward, then carry right to left to the next column. In simple first-grade work this orientation is not difficult. However, when more complex addition problems are introduced, he becomes confused by this new directionality which is backwards from the direction for reading and writing. To subtract or multiply, Paul must start at the bottom right, exactly opposite from the orientation for other paper/pencil work during the school day. In subtracting and multiplying he must work bottom to top, right to left. Long division involves a complex pattern of beginning left to right, then top to bottom, then bottom to top and right to left, then back to left to right again. If reading this description makes your head swim, you can imagine the confusion Paul faces when he is under pressure to hurry through arithmetic computation. He constantly loses direction and is forced to start over. When he is not given enough time to correct his directionality, he becomes enormously frustrated and confused.

Poor comprehension of sequence. Visual dyslexics are generally handicapped in any situation that requires them to comprehend sequence. Students like Paul usually cannot remember the order of the alphabet, months of the year, days of the week, multiplication tables, or even the day, month, and year of their birth. Paul's parents and teachers have complained about his habit of forgetting to do chores or carry out a set of instructions. The problem is seldom one of laziness or rebellion on his part; he simply does not build mental images of things in sequence. His comprehension of household duties, as well as classroom tasks, is as scrambled as his perception of printed symbols. It is unfortunate that such children are regarded as irresponsible. The fact is they are confused.

Of the three forms of dyslexia commonly found in classrooms, visual dyslexia is the most easily corrected. Students like Paul can usually identify the separate sounds of speech. Visual dyslexics usually can learn phonics. The major handicap is the inability to build mental images of printed symbols in correct sequence or position. Through appropriate drills Paul can learn to interpret printed symbols accurately, although he will remain a slow reader all of his life. Gradually he can learn to identify sequence in his environment, thus reducing his conflict with what adults expect. His greatest enemies are pressure for speed and pressure for large quantities of work to be produced. If he is given proper allowances for his limitations, Paul can become a strong student; he can even achieve advanced scholastic standing. Many adults have gained remarkable success in spite of visual dyslexia.

Auditory Dyslexia. The most difficult form of dyslexia to correct is the inability to hear the separate sounds of spoken language. Auditory dyslexia has little to do with hearing ability. Most auditory dyslexics have normal hearing. The basic handicap is like being tone deaf to music. Because auditory dyslexics cannot identify small differences between vowel sounds or consonant sounds, they cannot connect speech sounds to printed letters. Consequently these students are very poor at spelling and writing. Traditional phonics instruction is almost meaningless to most auditory dyslexics. They simply cannot hear the variations of speech sounds. The rules of phonics and spelling do not make sense.

For example, Donna is handicapped by auditory dyslexia. The seriousness of her problem is seen most clearly when she must write without help from others. Without being aware of Donna's perceptual limitations, her teacher has chosen to give a dictation test. Speaking clearly and slowly, the teacher dictates: "What kind of celebration did the Pilgrims have to show their thankfulness to God?" Donna's task is to encode this sentence with no help from anyone else. As usual, Donna's teacher becomes annoyed when Donna asks for the fifth time that the sentence be repeated. This need for repetition is characteristic of auditory dyslexics who are never sure that they have heard correctly. As she struggles to write the sentence, Donna is acutely aware of her teacher's impatient frown. Under these conditions, this is the best the child can do: "What cid of selbarshun dind the Plegms hev too sow tere takfulnis too Gode?"

At her very best writing speed, Donna requires from 3 to 5 minutes to encode a simple dictated sentence. Before she can finish one item, her teacher moves on to the next. As usual, Donna completes only two or three of the 10 dictated sentences. Thus she has met failure again, something she has come to expect.

Poor test taking. Children like Donna are at a serious disadvantage in standardized testing. The two most widely used intelligence tests for placing children in special classes are the Wechsler Intelligence Scale for Children–Revised (WISC-R) and the Stanford-Binet Intelligence Scale. These tests involve careful listening, accurate interpretation of what is heard, quick understanding of what is heard, then good explanation of certain information asked for by the examiner. Auditory dyslexics seldom score well on these verbal tests. Children like Donna usually comprehend only 30% to 40% of what they hear the first time. If the examiner is forbidden by the test administration instructions from repeating or saying items in simpler terms, Donna is stuck with only partly understood auditory concepts. She is left to guess, say nothing, or panic, depending upon her disposition. It is incredibly embarrassing to be an auditory dyslexic. Only part of what the person hears makes sense, especially on standardized tests. Donna almost never gets the point of oral situations as quickly as her peers. She sits isolated inside invisible walls feeling "dumb." Many auditory dyslexics develop cover-up behaviors that greatly irritate adults who do not understand the reason why the person acts silly or gives strange or irrelevant responses to oral statements.

Other problems. An auditory dyslexic is also handicapped in naming rhyming words, interpreting diacritical markings, applying phonics rules, and pronouncing words accurately. Because she does not hear differences between similar vowel sounds, Donna cannot tell the difference between *big* and *beg,* unless she hears the words used in context. One of the earmarks of auditory dyslexia is garbled pronunciation of familiar words.

For example, Donna is asked to read aloud the following passage from her science book:

> To test for acidity, place one teaspoon of bicarbonate of soda in a beaker. Measure one-fourth cup of vinegar, then pour slowly over the soda. Be sure not to use an aluminum cup.

Because she does not connect sounds to letters accurately, Donna reads aloud:

> To test for a-kye-da-ty, place one tee-poon of bi-kair-nate of soda in a braker. May-zer one-for cup vigener, then pore slow over the soda. Be sure not to use alunumum cup.

This tendency toward garbled speech is called *echolalia*. This tongue twisting constantly embarrasses Donna. She does not understand why others laugh at her tongue twisters.

Auditory dyslexia is difficult to correct because the person is cut off from hearing the letter/sound connections that constitute literacy. It is possible to devise drills and exercises for students like Donna, but this remedial work requires enormous patience on the part of both the teacher and student. As a rule, auditory dyslexics must devise their own sight-memory systems for coping with spelling and writing.

Many intelligent dyslexics have mastered common spelling patterns through mnemonic (memory) techniques. For example, Donna has learned to spell *then* and *when* correctly by remembering: "*Then* is *hen* with *t* in front; *when* is *hen* with *w* in front." Generally, the most effective teaching procedure for auditory dyslexia involves "word families," or spelling patterns. When similar patterns are studied together, Donna can memorize enough to satisfy ordinary writing requirements.

Dysgraphia. A third type of dyslexia is the inability to coordinate hand and finger muscles to write legibly. Many bright dyslexics have been seriously misjudged because their teachers could not read their writing. The work of extremely dysgraphic students actually resembles "chicken scratching," with few recognizable letters or words on the page. Often these disabled students fill page after page with scribbling in order to appear busy. Frequently they can read their own writing, although no one else can. It is difficult for dysgraphic students to learn to write legibly, although certain handwriting drills can increase the legibility of their work. Usually these students can learn to type and write with a word processor. Keyboard writing lets them communicate well in printed form.

Most cases of dysgraphia involve partly legible handwriting. Such writing is often quite small with many poorly formed letters. Many dysgraphics, however, write large with awkward, broken letters. The most effective teaching attitude is to help the dysgraphic student strive for legibility, not perfection. As with other dyslexics, dysgraphic students cannot handle pressure and speed. Any effort by adults to make these students hurry results only in frustration and increasingly poor self-concept.

Dyslexia in the Classroom

Rarely does a student exhibit just one form of dyslexia. Visual dyslexia is usually accompanied by auditory dyslexia, which complicates the teacher's task. If dyslexia is to be overcome, it must be identified early in a child's school experience. Time is a critical factor in solving perceptual disabilities. Follow-up studies of dyslexic students who have been treated at our center since 1973 show a rather somber pattern. If dyslexia is diagnosed before the child enters third grade, there is approximately 80% chance that the child can overcome his or her confusion with language symbols well enough to do satisfactory school work. If the condition is not diagnosed until fifth grade, there is approximately 40% chance of overcoming the handicap. For dyslexics who reach seventh grade before treatment is begun, there is only about 5% chance for enough correction to let the student reach grade level skills in writing and reading. Obviously, the hopes for successful remediation when the problem is not found until adulthood are small. When the symptoms are recognized early, much can be done within the regular classroom to overcome these handicaps.

2

Overcoming Visual Dyslexia

Within the dyslexic struggle to learn to read, spell, write, and do good math computation, a specific type of struggle is seen in many students. This is a particular kind of problem related to interpreting what the student sees in printed or written materials. What he or she sees is not correctly interpreted by the visual centers of the brain. Visual dyslexia has nothing to do with the eyes, although a majority of these strugglers have poor central vision, which was described in Chapter 1. Visual dyslexia refers to the tendency to reverse or rotate symbols, as well as to scramble the sequence of printed or written symbols.

Visual Dyslexia Syndrome

As described in Chapter 1, visual dyslexia refers to the inability to interpret printed symbols accurately. Many theories have emerged to explain this mysterious tendency for intelligent students to reverse letters and numbers, turn them upside down, or scramble the sequence of details. In the early 1900s an amazing theory speculated that little boys who get things backwards are victims of penis envy, a Freudian concept that seems to have little bearing upon visual processing. Another prevalent idea has been that poor teaching methods are responsible for symbol turning and confusion. Many professionals have speculated that some part of the brain must be "blind" to printed symbols, thus fostering the concept of "word blindness." The pioneering research of Norman Geschwind and his colleagues finally gave us the answer to the question: "Why do certain students get symbols backwards, upside down, or scrambled out of sequence?" Neurological research of the past decade has uncovered the fact that visual dyslexia occurs in a specific area of the left brain. The neuronal pathways that interconnect the visual cortex where the brain interprets what the eyes see on the page with the language centers where word meanings are processed do not make good enough connections. These brain pathways are not able to connect sounds to letters accurately or remember which way symbols should turn. Visual dyslexia occurs when certain left brain areas cannot process symbols correctly.

There is always danger in oversimplifying a complex idea. The human brain is obviously much more complex that a simple diagram or definition would show. But generally speaking, the visual cortex at the back of the brain is the major center where visual information related to reading, copying, and recognizing math symbols is processed. It is the job of the left brain hemisphere to master most of the concepts of formal education. The right brain is the picture brain. The right brain processes such functions as space, size, shape, color, texture, and form. The right brain recognizes faces and objects and how we represent our world through art and music and dance. The left brain has the task of learning to read from books, write information on paper, listen to oral information, learn new vocabulary, remember vast quantities of facts over a period of time, and earn educational diplomas and degrees. To become literate, one must have strong left brain skills. Dyslexia is a left brain deficit that makes it difficult or impossible to process classroom information that depends upon rapid interpretation of printed symbols, comprehension of oral language, and long-term memory for the myriad facts our culture regards as important.

Visual dyslexia is not caused by poor vision. A great deal of misinformation has been spread about how the eyes cause dyslexia. This mistaken notion says that if a student's vision can be corrected, dyslexia will go away. Many parents have spent a great deal of money for visual therapy and expensive glasses in the mistaken notion that visual correction will clear away their child's dyslexic problems. The eyes do not cause dyslexia. As was explained in Chapter 1, many dyslexics do have poor vision. But poor vision does not cause dyslexia. Correcting vision problems does not remove the dyslexic patterns that block reading, spelling, and handwriting.

Visual dyslexia occurs when the visual cortex cannot learn the correct orientation of printed symbols. Visual dyslexia involves getting certain symbols backwards (*b–d, p–q, 3, 5, 7, Z, S, L*). Visual dyslexia also involves turning symbols upside down (*M–W, n–u, 6–9, p–b*). Visual dyslexia frequently causes parts of words to be reversed (*brid/bird, gril/girl, sruprise/surprise*). Occasionally visual dyslexia causes whole words or number units to be read backwards. We call this *mirror image* (*on/no, saw/was, 81/18*). Some visual dyslexics scramble the order of what they see, as when a student says "four hundred ninety-one" when he or she sees *941*. This kind of printed symbol confusion occurs within specific areas of the left cerebral cortex. It is a brain-based dysfunction. It is not caused by carelessness or lack of trying. In fact, most visual dyslexics work very hard but cannot control this inadvertent scrambling, reversing, or rotating of details.

There is no single pattern that establishes dyslexia. Most children go through stages of faulty visual perception before they mature. Most preschool youngsters write letters and numbers backwards. Early readers often hold the book upside down before they learn to "turn it over." Before visual dyslexia can be confirmed, a definite set (syndrome) of behaviors must be identified. Only when an unmistakable cluster of perceptual disabilities is seen can anyone safely conclude that a person is dyslexic. The following sections contain descriptions of symptoms to look for when identifying visually dyslexic students. A checklist of specific deficits can be found in Appendix 1.

Confusion with Sequence

The underlying flaw in visual dyslexia is the student's inability to comprehend order or sequence. Few adults realize how much of the school day is geared to thinking according to the following model:

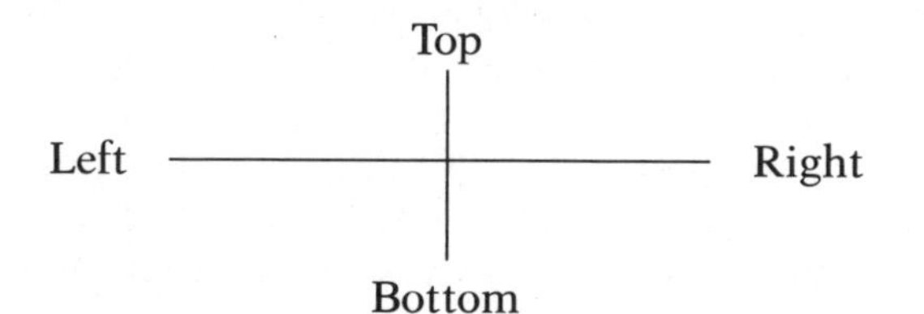

All reading, except for special instances in certain content areas, must be done left to right from the top to the bottom of the column or page. This principle is so commonly taken for granted that parents or teachers seldom mention it above the primary grades. It is assumed that anyone who reads will automatically go left to right and top to bottom. Unfortunately, this is not so for dyslexics.

The dyslexic orientation is just the opposite, or partly so. The dyslexic tendency is mirror image, meaning that the student's nature is to process symbols backwards (right to left and bottom to top). In fact, one of the developmental milestones we look for in kindergarten pupils is the point at which they "turn it over" and begin to think in terms of left to right and top to bottom. Approximately 80% of the student population learns this standard left-to-right, top-to-bottom orientation successfully, although late maturing children may not do so until second or third grade. The remaining 20% never fully achieve this standard orientation. Most of them are dyslexic.

Unfortunately for Paul, his primary teachers did not understand his difficulty with directionality. When the reading teacher introduced the letter *d*, she assumed that all of her pupils perceived it left to right (ball first, then the stick) and top to bottom (stick pointing up from the ball). Paul was completely unaware of his different orientation. He perceived the *d* right to left (stick first, then the ball) and bottom to top (stick below the ball). What the teacher perceived as *d*, Paul perceived as *p*. Several critical symbols are often misperceived by dyslexic learners: *d–b–p–q, M–W, u–n, 7–L, 6–9, h–y*. When dyslexics only partly rotate symbols, they often confuse *N–Z* and *3–M–W*.

The unfortunate consequence is that Paul is constantly told he is wrong. Unless someone explains how his perception differs, he enters the reading and writing process with no idea that he is heading the wrong direction up a very busy street. This is why he constantly collides with oncoming traffic. His teachers and most of his peers are proceeding in one direction while he travels the opposite or partly opposite way. So long as this situation is not recognized and understood, there is no way he can master the symbol system without constant conflict and the put-down of always being wrong.

Generally, this disability emerges whenever the visual dyslexic tries to deal with time, sequence, or details in a certain order. For example, instead of recalling an orderly progression of experiences over a period of time, Paul's memory of early childhood is a jumbled collection of events that do not fall into an orderly time sequence. In his perception of time, a broken arm 2 months ago happened right after he badly bruised his elbow when he was 3. Grandmother's death 5 years ago seems like last month to him.

Most children have a confused memory of their early years, but those with normal ability to sequence learn to connect their experiences in a time frame as they mature. Visual dyslexics seldom do. Since mastery of reading depends upon remembering letters in the right sequence, this learning disability is the greatest obstacle facing the visual dyslexic in today's curriculum.

Confusion with sequence is a major problem in Paul's trouble accepting responsibility. Because of his general frustration with order and sequence, he is continually in conflict with adult demands. At home his parents have given him the following responsibilities to be done each weekday morning: 1. Make bed before breakfast. 2. Brush teeth after breakfast. 3. Feed and water pets before catching school bus. 4. Take all homework back to school for day's classwork.

In the afternoon Paul faces another set of responsibilities: 1. Empty trash on Monday, Wednesday, and Friday. 2. Feed and water pets every afternoon. 3. Attend Cub Scouts on Tuesday afternoon. 4. Sweep garage on Saturday. 5. Read Sunday school lesson before bedtime on Saturday. 6. Pick up toys and tools from yard before noon on Saturday. 7. Bathe dog either Saturday or Sunday afternoon. 8. Be bathed and ready for bed by 9:00 each night.

These adult expectations have never been put into a written outline or on a calendar for Paul. His parents have told him these routines orally, assuming that he perceives time and sequence as clearly as they do. Paul's dyslexic tendencies to scramble the order of things leave him with an unstructured mass of responsibilities. In spite of his intentions to obey his parents, he finds himself confused and frustrated. As chores remain undone, adults conclude that the boy is lazy, stubborn, insubordinate, or forgetful. In reality, Paul is filled with dread and self-defeat. He has no way to communicate his dilemma to the adults who are obviously displeased with him. His unfinished chores generate family friction and almost constant misery for the child. After this kind of situation has gone uncorrected for several years, he has indeed become insubordinate and hostile. By the time he enters middle school he is convinced that he is worthless and incapable of success.

Similar frustration occurs in the classroom between teachers who do not understand and confused students like Paul. With many students to care for, the teacher naturally assumes that her instructions to Group A have been clear. As she turns to Group B, she is annoyed to see Paul not following her directions. Again the dyslexic student has failed in his relationships with the adult world. Since he cannot communicate his confusion to the teacher, she usually rejects him as being lazy, careless, or insubordinate. Thus the adult has unwittingly set the stage for misbehavior and unhappiness. Paul's failure to follow class instructions is due to perceptual difficulty in comprehending sequence, not willful disobedience.

In the classroom an alert teacher can identify confusion with sequence as students work with tasks involving series. For example, dyslexics like Paul are usually fluent in giving oral reports and carrying on conversations. Casual listeners are usually impressed by his stock of information and the concepts he gleans through listening and observation. There is, however, a noticeable flaw in his oral performance. He has difficulty recalling the correct sequence of details.

Many visual dyslexics cannot remember the day, month, and year of their birth. The teacher can check for this tendency through informal conversation in the room. Although he may know reams of statistics about his favorite ball team, Paul will usually stumble when asked to tell his full birth date.

Visual dyslexics also have trouble naming the days of the week and the months of the year. When asked to write this information, Paul keeps track by tapping his fingers, whispering a rhyme, or singing a song. In arithmetic he has an enormous struggle learning the multiplication tables; long division; how decimals, fractions, and percent correspond; mental computation involving money and measurement; and similar kinds of number skills.

Figure 2.1 and Figure 2.2 are examples from the Jordan Written Screening Test for Specific Reading Disability (JWST) (Jordan 1977, 1988b). This illustrates a visual dyslexic student's struggle to write and recall familiar details in sequence. Teachers and parents not only gain quick insight into sequence failure, but adults also begin to see evidence of dysgraphia and auditory dyslexia, if these disabilities also exist.

Another informal estimate of Paul's comprehension of sequence is to ask him to repeat a series of numbers. For example, he listens as the teacher says "*6-8-7-9-2.*" Then the teacher observes his efforts to repeat the numbers in the same sequence. Visual dyslexics usually fail in this kind of serial task. Or Paul might listen to a sentence and then try to repeat it verbatim: "Three men raced down the hill to their boat in the river." Dyslexics usually omit complete phrases or substitute different words. Frequently, they lose the theme of the sentence entirely.

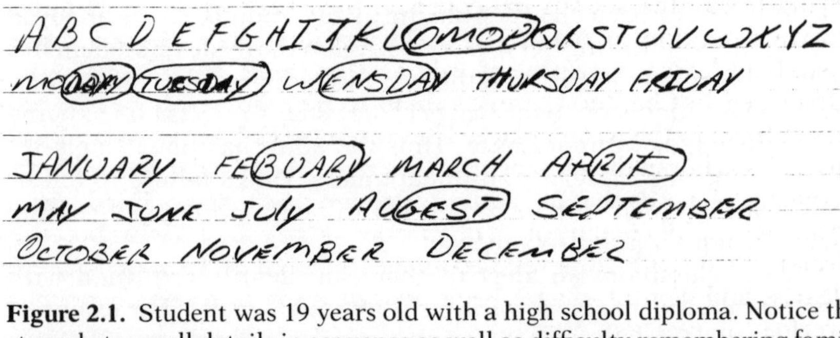

Figure 2.1. Student was 19 years old with a high school diploma. Notice the struggle to recall details in sequence as well as difficulty remembering familiar spelling patterns.

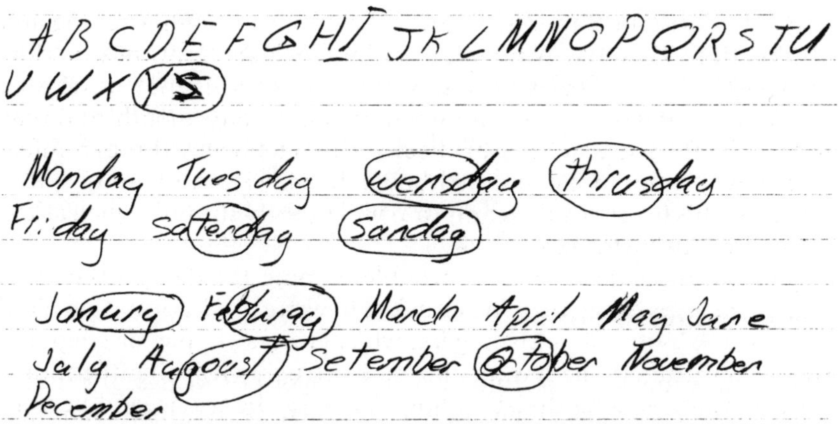

ABCDEFGHI JKLMNOPQRSTU
VWXYS

Monday Tuesday wensday thrusday
Friday saterday Sanday

Janury Feburay March April May Jane
July Augoust Setember October November
December

Figure 2.2. Student was 27 years old with a high school diploma. He had attempted several hours of college study before giving up trying to earn a college degree.

Faulty Reading Comprehension

Faulty perception of sequence is a major reason for Paul's poor performance on reading comprehension tests. Although a majority of students exhibit inferior comprehension to some degree, visual dyslexics are especially poor at retaining information that is presented in sequence. They must also deal with poor central vision in reading, which is described in Chapter 1. As these students read line after line, several problems begin to interfere with their understanding of what their inner voice is saying from the page. First, most visual dyslexics cannot maintain a smooth, forward rhythm in sounding out words in sentences. They literally take two steps forward, then one step back. If they read orally, they start to say the next word, stop, get stuck trying to say the sounds in sequence, then back up to try it again. Forward motion in reading is awkward and jerky. Second, many visual dyslexics transpose words as they read. Peripheral vision (described in Chapter 1) causes them to pick up words nearby and insert them in the wrong place. They often pull a later word back and insert it earlier in the sentence. As they read, they tend to scramble the sequence of words that are actually printed on the page. Third, visual dyslexics rapidly reach points of burnout as they read. Vision becomes overstressed, with the eyes becoming too tired to keep on focusing clearly, and mental images begin to fade away as a certain point of overload is reached. Many dyslexics cannot continue to read effectively longer than 3 to 5 minutes without taking a break. Some are able to read for 10 minutes before burnout occurs. Occasionally, a more mature dyslexic can read for half an hour before he or she must lay the book aside to rest. When all of these factors are considered, it is very difficult for visual dyslexics to read effectively, especially if they must hurry. They are forced to touch the print with a finger or pencil while they whisper to themselves over and over. This is a slow, tedious, time-consuming process that cannot be speeded up without triggering many more errors in decoding and comprehension.

Conservation of Form

The pioneering work of Inhelder and Piaget (1974) has given us a simple yet profound framework within which we may understand the growth of logic in children. Their term *conservation of form* is especially helpful in understanding the dyslexic learning disability. Conservation of visual form refers to the ability to see specific forms (letters, numerals, words, or shapes), then hold those mental images intact after the model is taken away. The act of reading could be described this way. As readers see visual forms on the printed page, their memory systems are expected to make lasting impressions which they use later after the book has been put aside or after their eyes have left a particular point of focus. Visual dyslexics cannot perform this perceptual act successfully. Students like Paul do not conserve the form. Once the model is no longer in view, the mental image is quickly lost, or parts of it are lost. Dyslexic readers conserve only bits and pieces of the whole model they have seen. In addition to conserving only part of the whole, students reverse or scramble the sequence of the parts. Severely dyslexic students cannot conserve form for more than a few seconds (very short-term memory). The moment their eyes move away from single words or parts of words, the mental image is lost or scrambled. Reading comprehension is especially difficult and tedious. Sometimes it is impossible to achieve.

Transformation

Conservation of form also involves the ability to change form (transformation). For example, in changing a statement into a question, the reader must hold the author's meaning (conserve the form) well enough to restructure the order of the words. Teachers of language arts can testify how difficult it is to teach dyslexics this operation in building variations of sentences. Reversibility is at the heart of arithmetic computation, especially when students must deal with such linear forms as ____ + 5 = 9. Students will be totally confused by math unless they can transform this linear visual pattern into:

$$\begin{array}{r} 5 \\ + \\ \hline 9 \end{array}$$

As he reads or listens, Paul does not develop or hold onto complete mental images of what he is reading or hearing. Just as he does not perceive an orderly sequence of time, neither does he comprehend the organization of an author's writing. When asked specific recall questions about his silent reading, Paul cannot retrieve enough organized information to respond the way adults expect. This constant failure to comprehend creates a dread of reading early in the visual dyslexic's school experience.

This handicap is especially troubling when Paul is asked to draw inferences or arrive at conclusions quickly. Standardized reading tests that require the student to read paragraphs and then answer questions within a strict time limit are almost impossible for dyslexics to do well. When given ample time, students like Paul often can arrive at satisfactory answers through trial and error or through the process of eliminating wrong answers. But timed pressure to hurry only increases the comprehension mistakes that frustrate visual dyslexics under the most relaxed study conditions.

Teachers complain about Paul's tendency to guess on pressure tests. Skipping down the page, marking answers at random, or refusing to check back over his work for errors are perfectly reasonable responses in view of his dyslexic handicap. By the time Paul has experienced several years of failure to comprehend what he reads, there is actually little else for him to do but guess. This is especially true when he is told that no consideration will be made for his slow pace, which is the only speed at which he can succeed.

Difficulty with the Alphabet

One of the major concerns of primary teachers is the visual dyslexic's inability to cope with the alphabet. The unstructured way in which the alphabet is introduced to primary pupils is largely to blame for uncorrected visual dyslexia. For the past 50 years teachers have not taught the alphabet in sequence to beginner pupils. We have known for years that beginners have been learning the alphabet sequence on their own from charts displayed in the classroom. Educators have generally discouraged direct teaching of the alphabet sequence before second grade.

This unstructured approach has posed no problem for most children. Youngsters with normal perception usually learn the alphabet as they need it. However, not teaching the alphabet in sequence has denied dyslexic children the only way of learning in which they can succeed—that of a structured, direct encounter with details in sequence. Since the visual dyslexic's principal weakness is faulty perception of sequence, having little or no sequence to follow proves disasterous when he or she is confronted with printed symbols. Had Paul been well grounded in the alphabet sequence at the very beginning of his school experience, he could have handled beginning reading tasks more successfully.

A simple technique for determining a student's perception of the alphabet is for the teacher to watch the student write it on ruled paper. Any dyslexic tendencies will quickly become apparent. Students with normal perception usually write the alphabet in sequence without hesitation. Visual dyslexics cannot.

When asked to write the alphabet, Paul will often stall, asking whether he should print or "write cursy." When told that it does not matter, he may want to know if he should use big or little letters. Dyslexic students seldom comprehend the terms *capital* and *lowercase.* Next Paul may ask whether he should go across or down the page. When finally at work, he will reach a stalling point, often at letter *M.* Whenever he bogs down, he goes back to *A* and whispers the letters one by one, trying to remember the whole sequence. Occasionally he will hum the alphabet song to himself. The observer can easily note the dyslexic's problem of synchronizing speech with writing. Paul's voice will usually be ahead of his eyes or finger. Consequently, reviewing his written work still does not help him identify errors.

Paul is very slow as he writes or prints the alphabet. The letters *m, n, p, u,* and *v* are often in scrambled positions. In addition to this sequence problem, he often confuses similar letters, such as *b–d–p–q, r–h–u–n, h–p–y, t–f–j, M–W, N–Z, r–s, v–w–k–y–x,* and *o–e–c.*

As he writes, Paul makes circular letters with backwards pencil motions. He frequently writes circular parts of letters with a clockwise motion, as well as marking from the bottom upward when writing *t, f, p, g, b,* or *d.* Unless the teacher is carefully observing his work, she might not be aware of this backwards motion, an earmark of dyslexia.

It is common for the visual dyslexic to mix capital and lowercase letters when writing the alphabet, as well as mixing manuscript and cursive styles. Paul's reasons for this inconsistent writing are actually quite practical. Because he has not been taught the sequence of the alphabet, he has never encountered the letters in relation to each other. He has devised his own system for identifying certain letters. Capital *B* and *D* are stable in his memory, although they may be written backwards, but lowercase *b* is too easily confused with *d, p,* or *q*. So long as he continues to deal with isolated letters in manuscript style, there is no dependable structure to which Paul can anchor his perceptions of the alphabet.

Figure 2.3 illustrates the kind of struggle many visual dyslexics have writing the alphabet and numbers from memory. It is unfortunate that well-meaning adults often misinterpret such handicapped work as the mark of inferior intelligence or laziness. These students struggle very hard to produce even this quality of work. Like Paul, the girl who wrote this was doing her best.

For further insight into a student's perception, the adult traces symbols on the student's back. Then the student writes what he or she "saw." The student may write in cursive when the adult has traced in manuscript. No issue should be made of this, however. The purpose of tracing on the back is to identify the student's immediate mental image of symbols, not to test his or her recognition of writing style. Figure 2.4 illustrates this technique of writing symbols on the student's back, then having the student write what he or she perceived.

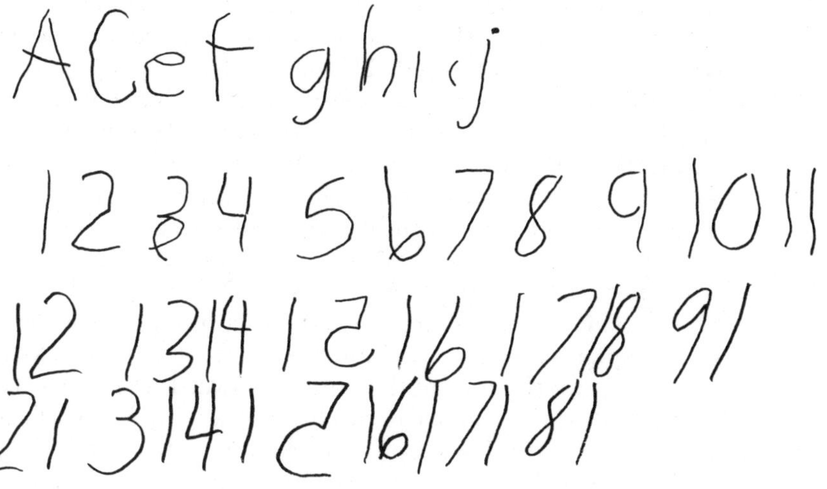

Figure 2.3. Writing sample from a female, age 8 years, 7 months. She struggled 15 minutes to write the alphabet and numbers 1 through 20. As she wrote 19, she completely lost her memory of number sequence. All teen numbers were written with the second numeral first, then 1 placed in front of the second numeral.

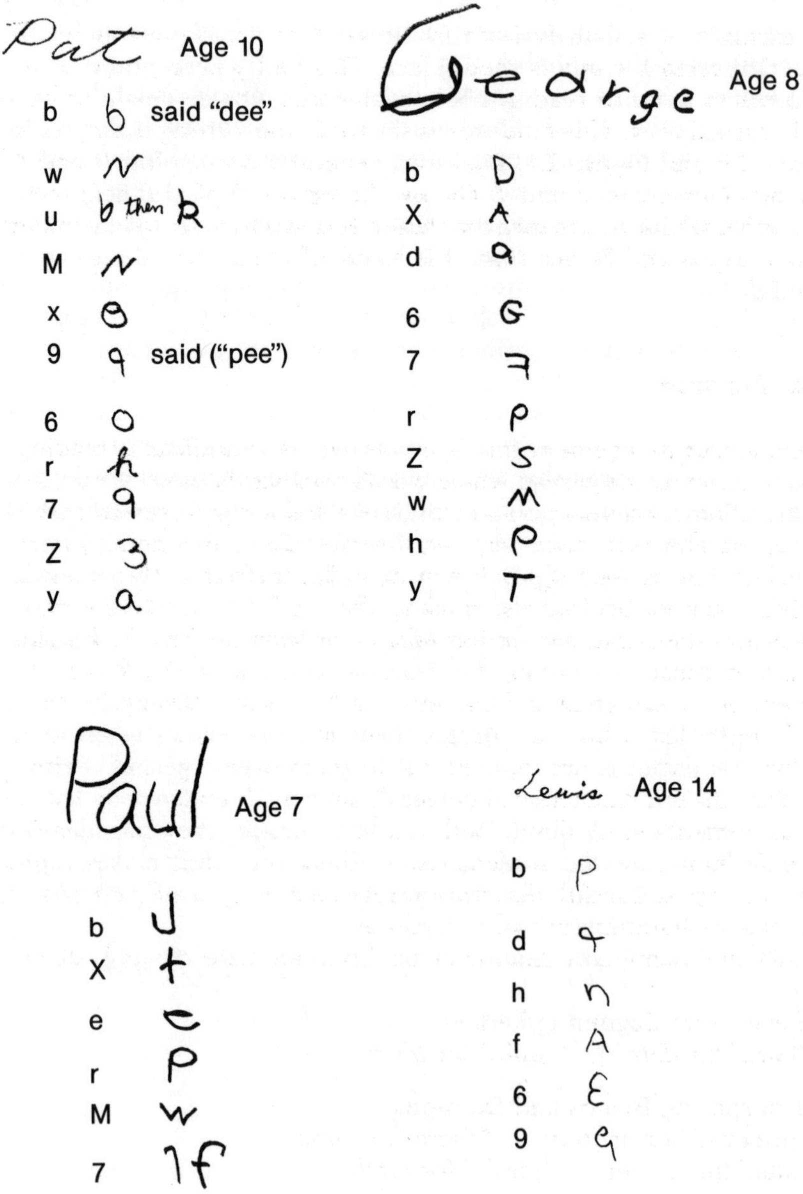

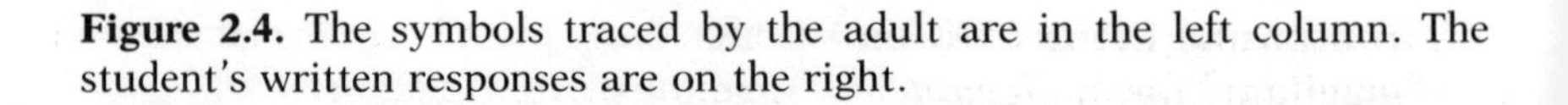

Figure 2.4. The symbols traced by the adult are in the left column. The student's written responses are on the right.

Reversal of Symbols

An earmark of visual dyslexia is the student's confusion as to the direction certain symbols should face. This faulty perception causes students to write or read symbols backwards, upside down, or partially turned over. This tendency is shown in the writing examples in Figure 2.5 and Figure 2.6. Dyslexics generally use capital *B* and *D* instead of lowercase *b* and *d*. The two humps on capital *B* help them remember which way to turn that letter. It is much easier to remember which way *B* and *D* face than it is to recall the correct direction of *b* and *d*.

Oral Reading

The tendency to reverse or turn symbols over is a handicap in reading. Visual dyslexics often read whole words backwards (*saw* for *was, but* for *tub*). Sometimes only certain kinds of syllables are reversed within words (*bran* for *barn, form* for *from, sliver* for *silver*). Beginning letters, especially lowercase *b, d, p, q, h, r, m, w,* and *u,* are frequently perceived upside down or backwards, causing the reader to mistake certain words for others that are similar (*daddy* for *baby, dark* for *bark*). This results in nonsense, forcing the dyslexic reader to go back over the context of the sentence to figure out what is wrong. Visual dyslexics can usually learn how to correct these reversal errors when their backwards patterns are pointed out to them over a period of time.

Parents and teachers can detect this reversal tendency by listening as students read aloud. Within a few minutes they can identify reversal habits. As the student reads aloud, the adult makes rapid notes of errors. Careful observation reveals any dyslexic patterns in the reader's handling of word elements.

The following oral reading errors often indicate visual dyslexia:

1. Reversal of Beginning Letters
   "bark" for *dark*   "dump" for *bump*

2. Transposing Blends and Digraphs
   "preform" for *perform*   "there" for *three*
   "star" for *stream*   "porfit" for *profit*

3. Substituting One Letter for Another
   "sleep" for *sheep*   "come" for *came*

4. Transposing Letters Within Words
   "magilant" for *malignant*   "macilous" for *malicious*

5. Reversal of Whole Words
   "on" for *no*   "saw" for *was*   "but" for *tub*
6. Failure to See Small Details (This includes habitual failure to see punctuation marks.)
   "house" for *horse*   "with" for *wish*
   "butter" for *better*   "hungry" for *hunger*
7. Omission of Endings
   "ever" for *every*   "her" for *here*   "happen" for *happened*
8. Telescoping
   "standarize" for *standardize*   "consently" for *consequently*
   "sudly" for *suddenly*
9. Perseveration
   "hopenen" for *hope*   "sudendely" for *suddenly*
   "farmerer" for *farmer*

Dyslexia is suspected only when several of these symptoms exist in the student's oral reading. Teachers must be careful to distinguish between poor vision and dyslexia (see Chapter 1).

Errors in Copying

It is especially hard for dyslexics to copy from the chalkboard or from a projection screen. This involves conservation of form, also called vision-to-motor transfer. The student must see the forms clearly, hold them intact in mental images (conserve the form) as he or she refocuses to the writing space, translate what was seen into specific motor movements (fine motor control), space it properly on the writing paper (figure-ground control), and end up with a legible resemblance to what was on the chalkboard or in the textbook. Busy teachers often forget what a complex task copying really is. It is a monumental task for dyslexics, who cannot conserve form without enormous concentration and effort. The use of over- head projectors has increased the pressure on many dyslexic students to take notes while the teacher lectures. The basic problems with symbol confusion force dyslexic students to work slowly. If they try to hurry, they quickly become frustrated trying to keep details in correct sequence.

Parents and teachers can rather easily identify which students are handicapped in copying. Students are asked to copy a paragraph from across the room. As they work at copying, the teacher watches for these tendencies:

1. Losing the place on the board
2. Erasing frequently

Dictated by Teacher		**Paul's Dyslexic Responses**	
bad		3Bab	lowercase *d* reversed
bag		4Bag	
ball		5Ball	
bed		6Bed	lowercase *d* reversed on top of unneeded *e*
bell		7Bell	letter *l* made bottom to top
big		8Big	
bill		9Bill	letters *i* and *l* made bottom to top
body		10Boby	lowercase *d* reversed
bug		11Bug	letter *g* circled several times with backward strokes
dad	began to write capital *B*	12Dab	lowercase *d* reversed
did	began to write capital *B*	13BiD	
dog		14Dog	wrote *o* and *g* with backward strokes
doll		15Doll	wrote *o* with backward stroke

Figure 2.5. Dyslexic writing with reversed letters, backward strokes, and mixed capital and lowercase letters.

Bob and Dan

Bob and Dan saw Sam Watts on the dock. The three men stopped. "See the big ship?" asked Sam.

"Sure did," Dan and Bob said. "Must be a mile long."

Bob and Dan saw Sam was in a hurry. "Got to run," Sam said. "See you."

"Sure," said Bob and Dan. "See you, Sam."

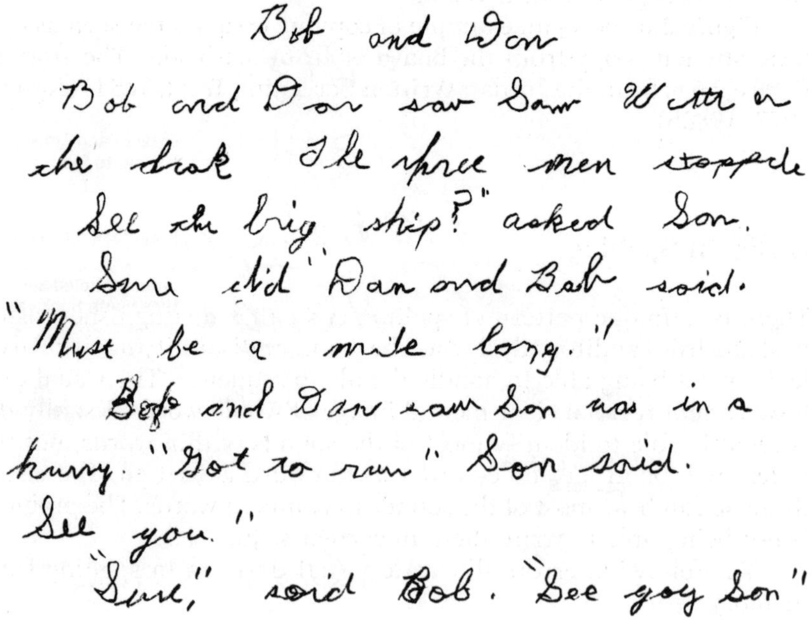

Bob and Dan

Bob and Dan saw Sam Wctta n
the duok The yprce men stoppde
See the big ship?" asked Son.
Sure did" Dan and Bab said.
"Must be a mile long."
Bop and Dan saw Son was in a
hurry. "Got to run" Son said.
See you."
"Sure," said Bob. "See goy Son"

Figure 2.6. Student was 14 years old. He needed 37 minutes to copy this story.

3. Overprinting to correct mistakes on paper
4. Misspelling on paper
5. Failing to observe capital letters
6. Failing to observe punctuation marks
7. Failing to space properly on paper
8. Reversing letters
9. Reversing whole words
10. Working unusually slowly

Dyslexic-like flaws can also be caused by certain types of defective vision (see discussion of vision problems in Chapter 1). Adults must be careful not to mistake dyslexic confusion with sequence and poor writing with poor central vision.

Figure 2.6 shows an example of copying errors often seen as dyslexic students copy from the board or from textbooks. The story in Figure 2.6 is from the Jordan Written Screening Test (JWST) (Jordan, 1977, 1988b).

Errors in Spelling

There is a unique pattern of spelling error that distinguishes visual dyslexia from auditory dyslexia. The primary disability in visual dyslexia is not being able to handle details in sequence. The visual dyslexic cannot recall a clear mental image of whole words. Usually the student is able to identify most of the sounds within words, but the letters will be in scrambled order as the word is written. The visual dyslexic can hear most of the sounds in common words. The problem is not being able to write them in correct sequence.

The following errors illustrate visual dyslexia in spelling from memory.

Word in Paul's mind	His written response
rode	roed
ate	aet
goes	gose
heaven	haveen
marriage	mirarage

Activities for Overcoming Visual Dyslexia

As every dyslexic adult will verify, it is not possible to overcome dyslexia completely. Some dyslexics gradually outgrow enough of the problem to become comfortable students in their late teens or early twenties (secondary dyslexia or developmental dyslexia). Some dyslexics do not outgrow their patterns even as adults (primary dyslexia). However, all dyslexics can master techniques to help them reduce the level of frustration and increase success with reading, writing, and math computation. New technologies are giving dyslexics remarkable ways to work around handicaps in spelling and writing. Each new generation of word processors provides more helpful ways to spot misspelled words and develop better sentence structure. As we have seen in Chapter 1, it is vitally important for dyslexia to be diagnosed early in the child's life so that remedial training can be started before years of failure have destroyed the child's will to try. The rest of this chapter presents certain concepts that are essential for dyslexics to master. If these concepts are taught carefully over an extended period of time, it is possible for most dyslexics to overcome enough of their handicap to succeed in formal education.

Teaching Time Sequence

Chapter 1 presented the diagram of how dyslexia varies from mild to severe. Visual dyslexics who struggle at Level 5 or higher have difficulty with time concepts. They do not automatically perceive how time passes in a given sequence. They live from moment to moment, day to day, week to week, month to month, and year to year without developing an overall view of how time passes in their lives. It is possible to teach dyslexics to think in terms of an orderly sequence of time if this training combines visual guidelines as well as continual talking about time.

The first step in establishing awareness of time sequence is to provide children with visible, tangible cue systems that show chronological order. In primary grades this is usually done with monthly calendars to teach the days of the week within the month. Few teachers present time in more that 1-month calendar units.

Dyslexic children must be drilled in the basic units of time: seconds and minutes, minutes and hours, hours and days, days and weeks, weeks and months, months and years, years and decades, decades and centuries. Busy adults usually bypass steps in this continuum, hopping from minutes and hours to days and weeks, omitting years, decades, and centuries altogether. Activities involving time concepts seldom build an unbroken, sequential awareness of time. Dyslexic youngsters seldom see the continuum from the smallest units (seconds) to largest units (centuries). Bright children without dyslexic tendencies soon figure out this time structure. But without visible, tangible models as constant reminders, dyslexics fail to perceive the order and units of time. This has crippling results in social studies (historical sequence), math (lapse of time), and science (seasonal change; geological classification). This basic deficit in time sequence leaves the dyslexic student unable to cope with many time situations that adults take for granted.

For example, every dyslexic child's classroom and room at home should have charts and calendars showing how time units move forward in relation to each other. These time flow charts should be displayed in sequence all year long. Dyslexics need to be involved every day in a review of time units: minutes, hours, days, weeks, months, years, seasons. Over a period of time this basic knowledge of time sequence begins to fall into place for them. In September school should begin with a visual model of how summer has merged into fall. Day by day the dyslexic student should see a visual progression involving such concepts as: during last summer, this fall, when winter comes, last week, now, next week, last month (August), this month (September), next month (October), how long until Thanksgiving (November), how long until Hanukkah or Christmas (December), and so forth. Dyslexics need a permanent display of this step-by-step presentation of time sequence in which nothing is left to chance. When this sort of carefully programmed sequence of time is done over a spread of time, adults see dyslexic youngsters beginning to grasp the concepts of chronological order. As birthdays, family events, and personal activities are displayed on this visual model of time, visual dyslexics begin to comprehend this knowledge of time sequence in our culture.

Creative parents and teachers will have no difficulty turning a wall into an effective, colorful time map for dyslexic youngsters. The great temptation is for adults to go back to their old habits of neglecting this sort of consistent perceptual training. Teachers tend to become sidetracked by pressure to "get through the books on schedule." Getting through the books is irrelevant for students who still have not mastered sequence. If adults can understand that some children will more than make up the pages in the books *after* the foundation has been laid, then it will be easier to be patient with the importance of daily attention to building concepts of time sequence.

At this point it is essential to ask: "What do these special children need?" If visual dyslexics need daily instruction in the fundamentals of chronological order, then getting through Unit Two of science or social studies is irrelevant. It is not a waste of time to do memory drill in order to master the days of the week or the months of the year in sequence. The ultimate goal of such drill is comprehension of how specific days and months fit together on the calendar. Before this level of practical understanding can be reached, however, dyslexics must spend many hours of drilling to name the days and months, as well as to write them from memory. It is a serious cultural deficit for an individual in the labor market to stumble over which day or which month it is. Instead of belaboring irrelevant textbook matter with dyslexic students, the teacher should spend that time establishing a solid working knowledge of time sequence, regardless of the age of the students involved.

Teaching Alphabet Sequence

For half a century American educators have thought themselves clever for concealing alphabet sequence until after children have learned to read. For most children this has done no harm, largely because bright youngsters have been learning the alphabet anyway from the model cards displayed above the chalkboard. Dyslexic children have not absorbed the alphabet because they cannot comprehend sequence presented in an indirect way. They are stymied when called upon to alphabetize words, find entries in the dictionary, or locate material in reference books. When the alphabet letters are doled out in random order, there is no point of reference by which the dyslexic student can comprehend where letters are within the alphabet sequence. This deficiency poses serious problems in upper grades.

Some teachers and parents must recover from guilt feelings implanted by recent educational tradition which taught them that rote memory drill is not correct. By virtue of their handicap, dyslexic students have no other choice than to memorize. If the alphabet sequence is to be mastered, it must be done through rote drill—day after day of toil, arranging movable letters in correct order, copying from models, and writing the sequence from memory. If the student has not learned the alphabet sequence, then it is irrelevant to struggle through higher level activities that rest upon such knowledge.

Beginner pupils should start learning the alphabet sequence by handling cutout three-dimensional forms. Creative teachers can devise their own alphabet models using clay, pipe cleaners, or hand-cut paper forms. It is unnecessary to spend precious funds on expensive materials to teach alphabet sequence. In fact, the simpler the models, the better they usually are for teaching purposes.

In mastering the alphabet, it is essential that dyslexic children learn only one major concept at a time. For this reason it is detrimental for a teacher to introduce phonic principles at the same time letter shapes are being mastered. Dyslexic children must not be expected to manipulate two forms of information at once during the initial stages of learning a new concept. For example, Paul should associate the names of the letters with their shapes, not the sounds for the letters. He should match the letter *A* with the name of the letter, but he should not be exposed to "phonics" until he has first learned the name of the letter. Sounds for letters should come after the sequence and shapes of the letters have been mastered.

Alert teachers will be able to tell when a child is ready for a more advanced level of experience in handling alphabet sequence. The following learning sequence shows the kinds of activities the dyslexic student should do:

Step One	Master alphabet sequence with movable letters
Step Two	Trace over alphabet sequence on chalkboard
Step Three	Trace over alphabet sequence on paper (or on plastic wipe-off sheets)
Step Four	Copy alphabet sequence at the chalkboard as student looks at model cards or teacher's written model)
Step Five	Copy alphabet sequence on lined paper as student looks at alphabet chart or teacher's written model
Step Six	Write alphabet sequence with model nearby so student can see it if he or she forgets
Step Seven	Write alphabet sequence from memory with no reversals, rotations, or letters out of sequence

Adults have made the mistake of rushing dyslexic children too fast through this developmental sequence. Today's kindergarten programs usually introduce Step One through Step Three of the above outline. Most schools assume that primary pupils have mastered all seven steps by the time they begin third grade. This is not the case, as revealed by thousands of high school students who cannot handle alphabet sequence from memory. The urgent need of dyslexic students is to master alphabet sequence, no matter how old the student is when the deficiency is discovered. It is irrelevant for students to struggle with book reports or themes until they have mastered the sequence of the alphabet.

Traditionally, cursive writing style has been postponed until third grade on the assumption that primary children need to learn the finger dexterity skills of manuscript print before advancing to the more complicated motor patterns of cursive style. This assumption has never been supported by research evidence. On the contrary, children who begin handwriting with cursive style seldom show disabling dysgraphic tendencies later in writing activities. Largely because of the consistent, flowing motor patterns established through cursive writing, alphabet sequence is quickly established when cursive style is introduced. For example, the D'Nealian handwriting program published by Scott, Foresman and Company is excellent for children who struggle with traditional "ball and stick" manuscript printing.

The quickest remediation of reversal and rotation tendencies in writing is quite simple. The teacher or parent writes a clearly legible line of alphabet letters, all connected in cursive style as if they were spelling one long word. Then the student practices tracing over the written model as the adult guides the wrist to establish proper hand movements. Over a period of a few weeks this kind of practice pays off generously. The dyslexic writer becomes increasingly self-confident at writing. His or her perception of alphabet sequence quickly develops, and the student becomes aware of where each letter is located within the alphabetic sequence. By having a dependable model as a guide, visual dyslexics find great security. Soon they are ready to start copying the adult's handwriting directly beneath the written model. In a few days or weeks they can write their own cursive sequence with only occasional reference to a model. For dysgraphic students the process of remediation is often slow and frustrating. However, cursive writing style is the most effective way to establish automatic knowledge of alphabetic sequence.

Comprehending Instructions

Trouble building complete mental images through listening to a flow of oral information involves the dyslexic learner with continual failure whenever adults give oral assignments. This inability to comprehend instructions widens the area of conflict to include classmates and other family members. When dyslexics fail to understand parents' or teachers' intentions regarding assigned activities, the whole family or class soon becomes involved in the argument.

Helping students pay attention to sequential steps in carrying out instructions is actually rather simple. Instead of forcing them to depend upon memory, the parent or teacher provides a simple written outline of what is expected. If the dyslexic student can read, a simple outline is provided, listing each step or each responsibility. This technique is especially suitable for routine work, such as daily chores or work schedules which stay the same from day to day. When clear written instructions are given in textbook or workbooks, the teacher has a ready-made visual aid in teaching how to follow sequence in interpreting instructions. Otherwise the teacher must make his or her own lists and outlines for the student to see.

Kindergarten and primary teachers often solve the problem by creating picture code systems, such as using animal pictures, colored shapes, or other easily interpreted markers as cues. Children who easily lose track can refer back to the chart to be reminded of what to do next.

Older dyslexics have the same basic needs for quick reference. As they listen to a series of directions, dyslexics start to lose the sequence of what is expected. Most adults are unaware of how complicated their oral directions actually are. For example, in getting her arithmetic class under way, a teacher in fourth grade will usually make 20 or more short statements. Children are adept at "tuning in" and "tuning out," so they seldom pay attention to everything the teacher says. They are expected to "filter" the teacher's flow of information.

For example, the teacher's instructions might sound like this:

> "Now class, it's time for arithmetic. Put away your social studies books and get out your arithmetic books. Tom, sit down. Yes, Mary? No, you don't need two pencils. Now, class, be sure you have your pencils ready. Open your workbooks to today's lesson. Yes, Joe? No, I didn't *say* get them out, but you know I meant for you to. Now, children, open your books to page 251. What, Sue? Yes, you may get a drink for your hiccups. Now, on page 251 we are ready to review short division. ..."

This steady flow of speech is supplemented by *paralanguage,* the unspoken gestures, facial expressions, variations of tone, and other nonverbal ingredients of group communication. Most children edit the running dialogue, tuning in only when the teacher or a fellow student says something important that must be remembered. A student without a listening handicap monitors the teacher's dialogue like this:

> "...It's time for arithmetic....Put away your social studies books...get out your arithmetic books...you don't need two pencils...open your workbooks to today's lesson...open your books to page 251...we are ready to review short division. ..."

Dyslexic listeners cannot do this kind of editing successfully. They cannot determine what the teacher thinks is essential because they cannot filter out the unnecessary information bombarding them from all sides. When there is no visual outline that lists the essential steps, the dyslexic student is lost. However, if the teacher has provided a written list for later reference, the student has a chance. By referring to the following outline on the chalkboard, Paul can cope with the teacher's expectations:

For Today's Arithmetic

1. Have one pencil ready.
2. Open textbook to page 251.
3. Open workbook to page 97.
4. For tomorrow do the 15 problems on workbook page 97.

Many teachers have found that it helps to record their daily instructions on tape. After the class is at work, those who did not understand the instructions can put on headphones and listen to the assignment in private, repeating the instructions as many times as needed. As a last resort, students can go to the teacher individually. When some kind of face-saving alternative is provided for dyslexics, the entire group is spared the arguments encountered when the same one or two students disrupt the learning atmosphere every day by clamoring for repeated explanations.

Failure to comprehend sequence in instructions is the primary cause for failure with arithmetic story problems, science experiments, and chronological order in social studies. Although outlining is often introduced in elementary grades, the purpose for making brief outlines is frequently not clear to the students. An essential skill for the dyslexic is being able to write down the essential ingredients of a problem step by step. Providing lists of instructions or tapes is one way of outlining what the adult expects of the child. Leaving the interpretation of commands up to the dyslexic student is not fair, unless the teacher has taken great pains to make things clear. The overwhelming need of dyslexics is for the adult to leave easily retraceable steps for them to follow. If the handicapped student has a written list of cues, he or she can learn to cope with most classroom expectations.

Correcting Reversals and Rotations

Teaching visual dyslexics not to turn things upside down or backwards is not always possible in a typical classroom setting. This tendency often requires a one-to-one teaching relationship, which few teachers can provide during the school day. However, certain remedial steps can be taken regardless of the teacher's time limitations.

Remediation must begin with honesty. This statement may seem strange to experienced teachers and parents who are above reproach in their personal ethics. However, adults seldom deal openly with problems involving learning disability. If a student is to find relief from brain-based learning disability, this must be dealt with openly. This does not mean that an adult would embarrass a student before the class. The approach required for successful remedial work with dyslexics is to show them the kinds of mistakes they make, and then develop a reminder system to help them monitor their work against such mistakes in the future.

In a quiet conference away from the prying eyes and ears of other students, the teacher should explain how the student's work has been analyzed for dyslexic characteristics. For example, the teacher should present a checklist of visual dyslexic characteristics (see Appendix 1). This simple list helps the adult explain in simple terms that the student does not "see" letters, numerals, or words like most people do. Many adults recoil from this sort of counseling on the grounds that it is cruel and risky to expose a person to such frank self-knowledge. The fact is that it is cruel *not* to explain to the handicapped student exactly what it is that produces conflict in the learning situation. Of course it might be foolish to tell an overly fearful child: "You are dyslexic." But if students are mature enough to ask what the problem is they should be told. Half of the success of remediating these tendencies depends upon the student's full cooperation. It is impossible to enlist their cooperation if students are not informed of the nature of the problems they are supposed to be correcting.

A teacher or parent will readily understand the need for honesty by recalling how adults feel when medical doctors withhold information during illnesses. Adults are quickly frightened when an examining physician mutters "Hmmmmmm!" or "Aha!" but never explains those reactions to the apprehensive patient. If teachers and parents can realize that children have the same needs to know what is going on, it will make remedial work with dyslexics much more effective.

Quietly, unemotionally, and openly the teacher or parent should point to specific examples of dyslexic confusion in the student's work, explaining that these are the reasons for low grades or criticism. The student should be told that he or she "sees some letters backwards or upside down." The adult should point out exact instances in assignments ("beb" for *bed;* "mnst" for *must*). Or the adult might play part of a tape to let the student hear his or her own voice invert syllables ("gril" for *girl;* "on" for *no*). Whatever the dyslexic tendencies are, the teacher or parent must explain them to the student, in whatever detail the student wishes. The teacher or parent must not be judgmental or condescending. If the conference can be conducted as a conversation between an interested adult and a student with a need, the result will be relief and a sense of understanding on the student's part. After all, he or she has known for a long time that something has been wrong. At last somebody is explaining it all in simple language.

Parents and teachers should encourage the dyslexic student to suggest ways for correcting the problem, especially in upper grades. Intelligent primary students are also able to have a voice in planning their remedial activities. The teacher must make it clear what the expectations are. This is often done in the form of a simple contract, which states the specific dyslexic problems and what the student promises to do each day to overcome them. The teacher must make it clear how much time can be given one-to-one during the school day. If the teacher can manage three 5-minute periods during recess or the lunch hour, this needs to be specified. The important thing is that the student know how much individual attention can be expected.

The most promising source of help for one-to-one tutoring during the school day is older students, volunteer teacher aides, or other individuals who can fit quietly into the school routine without disrupting classroom procedures. Older students are especially effective as tutors, provided there is no clash between them and the dyslexic child. A small amount of attention on a one-to-one basis goes a long way in building self-confidence in the dyslexic. Tutoring need not go on for hours to be effective. In fact, three 45-minute sessions during the school week are often enough to unlock the perceptual block, allowing the dyslexic to make significant progress in overcoming a specific problem.

Arithmetic. The perceptual dilemma dyslexic children face in mastering arithmetic skills is discussed briefly in Chapter 1. The major deficit is inability to change direction without becoming confused and losing the mental picture of the number relationships involved. Arithmetic computation above the primary level involves thousands of transformations as groups and number units change position within the problem. Arithmetic symbols represent highly condensed decoding (reading). A single symbol often stands for a complex abstract concept. It would take many lines of writing to express clearly the memory factors involved in most simple problems and equations. Students who tend to scramble sequence, lose direction, or reverse or transpose details find it very difficult to master the many variations they encounter beyond beginning computation levels.

The foremost consideration for parents and teachers to remember when working with dyslexics is to keep the structure as nearly the same as possible. It is distressing for dyslexics to have to shift back and forth from linear form (7 + _____ = 13) to vertical form:

$$\begin{array}{r} 7 \\ + \\ \hline 13 \end{array}$$

Lessons requiring students to change the form frequently from line to line impose so much memory stress that most dyslexics quickly become agitated or rebellious. Wise teachers who recognize memory and directional problems in their students keep the format of problems the same. Dyslexics are capable of learning linear form (equations), but they cannot rapidly change back and forth from one mode to another. Since the goal of education is to prepare students for future situations beyond the classroom, it is totally unimportant that all children change directionality quickly on demand, just for practice. Dyslexics need structure that stays the same as much of the time as possible. Whenever teachers must vary the problem form, dyslexic students must be given all the time and help they need in making the perceptual change. Some children never learn to do so at all. For them, the standard vertical problem form is essential, since this is the style they will need the most in their future lives.

An increasingly common practice is to let children use inexpensive pocket calculators for classroom computing. Dyslexics need to develop functional knowledge of paper and pencil computing, of course, but there is no way they can handle the quantity of work prescribed by most classroom programs. Paul cannot possibly work arithmetic problems faster than his usual plodding rate. His rate of thinking forces him to go slowly when he must translate mental images into writing. A hand calculator gives him an instant means of speeding up his work, and the increase in his self-confidence is just as rapid. With a calculator he can pour out arithmetic work along with the fastest pencil performers in the class. What a boost to his morale it is to hold his own after so much embarrassment and sense of failure.

High school and college math instructors make wide use of pocket calculators. In fact, the slide rule in math courses has long been obsolete. Forcing learning disabled students to labor with traditional paper and pencil computation is just as obsolete, especially when no real purpose is served except to satisfy tradition. "We've always done it this way" does not justify forcing dyslexics to agonize over memorized facts when a remarkably simple new technology is now available. The pocket calculator has come into its own as a valid educational tool. Adults who resist its use are refusing to step into the 21st century.

Finger Touching. Students with loose sensory integration have to do something physical to keep all of their memory circuits plugged in. They cannot develop or hold onto complete mental images just by thinking about numbers. They must touch/say/see all at the same time. Dyslexics who cannot do mental arithmetic without whispering and "counting their fingers" are crippled in typical math assignments if adults demand that they work silently with no finger involvement. A remarkably effective touch/see/say math program has been developed by a creative group of teachers in Colorado. The Touch Math program (published by Touch Math, P.O. Box 7402, Colorado Springs, Colorado 80933-7401) is excellent for establishing basic math skills with dyslexic children. Students are taught a system that incorporates several sensory pathways at the same time. This allows them to pull loose mental images together and to recall math information correctly. Students learn to tap fingers while whispering math facts. Touch Math is a greatly simplified form of the Chisanbop finger computation method taught for centuries in the Orient. Dyslexic students are greatly helped by this math system which teaches them to integrate their sensory pathways effectively.

Parents and teachers must keep two cardinal rules in mind when teaching arithmetic skills to dyslexic children:

1. *Keep the structure constant.* Because conservation of form (reversibility and transformation) is so difficult for dyslexics, arithmetic structure must remain the same from day to day. Frequent changes in format and directionality are devastating to confused students who cannot handle rapid shifts in form.

2. *Keep the work rate slow.* Dyslexics must not be pressured to hurry in computation. If quantity is important, then they must be given the bypass mode of a pocket calculator. A hand calculator is an equalizer, making up the vast difference between the perceptual endowments of rapid learners and the disabilities for which the dyslexic child is not responsible. If paper and pencil routines are essential, then the work rate must be slow. If calculators are permitted, then dyslexic students can produce as much arithmetic work as their peers.

Reading Orally. Reading aloud is essential for correcting reversals and rotations. As the dyslexic student reads slowly from one text, the tutor or teacher monitors from another copy. As mistakes occur, the monitor quietly says, "Look at that word again, Paul. How is it spelled?" This sort of cuing is low-key. There is no embarrassment or shame in calling Paul's attention to his errors. By immediately pinpointing error patterns, the tutor reinforces accurate symbol perception on a one-to-one basis. Intelligent dyslexics soon begin to catch their own errors by coordinating what they see, say, and hear.

Keyboard Writing. Most dyslexic students can develop outstanding writing skills if they are taught to work with a computer/word processor system that has a self-correcting spelling feature. Several word processor systems are now available that signal when words are misspelled. Within a few years word processors will also have self-correcting grammar and sentence structure programs, as well as programs that correct punctuation mistakes. This new technology will let dyslexic writers bypass most of their problems in producing written work. An excellent touch typing program is helping thousands of dyslexics become fluent with keyboard writing. The *Type-Write Program* (Johnson & Stetson, 1984; published by PRO-ED) was designed especially for dyslexic students, especially children. The first segment of the program teaches touch typing skills that correspond to the keyboards of standard typewriters and most microcomputers and word processors. Once students know which fingers go to which keys, they begin to type words, phrases, and spelling patterns that significantly increase language skills. By the time the student has finished the three-part *Type-Write Program,* much improvement has been achieved in spelling from memory, constructing sentences correctly, paying attention to left-to-right sequence, noticing all of the important details, and seeing how words are related in reading passages. All of the essential reading and writing skills are enriched by the *Type-Write Program.*

The goal for dyslexic students should be to do most of their necessary school writing with a word processor or typewriter by the time they enter fourth grade. This is especially important for dysgraphic students who cannot write large quantities legibly. Keyboard writing sets the student free to put thoughts and information onto paper without "shorting out" and losing so much of the mental image. The physical act of pinching the pencil (tactile pressure) "shorts out" the mental image. The quick act of tapping keys does not short out the mental image. Keyboard writing for the dyslexic/dysgraphic student sets the mind free for much more fluent expression of ideas and information. Once parents and teachers have accepted keyboard writing as a legitimate alternative for doing school work, much of the conflict over dyslexic writing disappears. An editor must still look over the finished writing to help the student spot mistakes, but keyboard writing lets dyslexic students become skilled with encoding far beyond the level they can achieve with pencil or pen. Becoming a skilled word processor develops amazing leaps of self-confidence and motivation for students who are crippled with traditional paper and pencil writing.

Using Tachistoscopes. Individual perceptual training is greatly enhanced through the use of tachistoscopes of various kinds. These devices range from simple handmade flash cards to expensive electronic instruments mounted in learning booths. The dyslexic student practices seeing whole words or phrases in a flash. He or she immediately tries to pronounce the word, and then writes or types it while the visual image is still fresh. Finally, the student flashes the pattern again to check for accuracy. This kind of forced response is highly effective in correcting faulty visual perception, particularly when reversal and rotation tendencies are involved.

Matching Word Forms. Daily drill activities can be devised by the parent or teacher to develop accuracy in word discrimination. A simple word is presented on a flash card. After a quick glance, the dyslexic student tries to find a matching word within a line of similar words. The following examples from the Jordan Written Screening Test (Jordan 1977, 1988b) show how this can be done:

Word on Card	**Choices on the Worksheet**
barn	barn pran puar buar narb uarp barn
spot	spot tobs tops stop stob sbot tobs
silver	sliver silver vilser rivils revlis selvir

Reading with a Marker. Chapter 1 includes a discussion of off-center vision in many dyslexic readers. For a majority of those with visual dyslexia symptoms, it is essential that the student use some kind of marker in order to read paragraphs, stories, and pages of print. Some dyslexics must use a card with a slot cut out so that only one or two words are seen at one time. Others need a card marker held just below each line as the eyes work across the line of print. Some visual dyslexics can get by with brushing a finger or a pencil eraser beneath each word as the eyes refocus from place to place along the line of print. Others must hold a marker below the line while the left thumb punches each word above the line. Still other students need to use two fingers to frame each word or isolate chunks within words. It does not matter what the student uses as a marker. Those of us who have taught literacy skills in store-front classrooms or in prison facilities have seen adults use cigarettes, pocket combs, sticks of gum, and other kinds of unusual markers. The point is that most dyslexics must develop some kind of marking system to hold their focus steady. Without marking, their eyes soon lose the place and they can no longer see printed details clearly. Reading with a marker usually doubles or triples the length of time a dyslexic person can read before he or she must rest from burnout.

Keeping Track of Progress. Parents and teachers who help a student conquer dyslexia usually keep track of progress. This should be a simple procedure, requiring a minimum of bookkeeping. Older students can learn to record their own progress, as they do in other individualized study programs at school. The initial task is for the adult to prepare a guide sheet, outlining the student's specific dyslexic tendencies. The checklists in this book provide a convenient basis for constructing the guide sheet. Brief comments should be recorded to indicate improvement. The final entry beside each dyslexic characteristic is the date when the problem has come under control. Of course it is impossible to know the very day when certain tendencies disappear. But the student and the instructor can compile a record of improvement, which is the major consideration in building self-confidence. This simple diagnostic record offers two advantages for remedial work at home or in the classroom. First, prescriptive teaching is quite simple, once the specific deficiencies have been identified on the checklist. This means that the teacher can pace the student's progress from one skill level to the next without too much frustration. Until the record sheet shows that a specific problem has been cleared up, the teacher knows not to push the student on to a more frustrating level of activity. Second, the record sheet forms the basis for a reasonable work contract between the child and the tutor. The dyslexic student knows exactly how much remains to be corrected in his or her learning behavior. Without this simple record and communication between teacher and child, everyone involved continues to wallow in frustration and failure.

The dyslexic student's frustration threshold is an accurate index to the success of remedial activities. So long as parents and teachers observe tension, disruptive behavior, frustration, anxiety, dread, avoidance tactics, and other symptoms of learning difficulty, they know that the student's learning disabilities remain operational. Regardless of the age of the student or the lateness in the year, it is useless and dangerous to push the dyslexic further and further on through the books. Adults will know when the perceptual foundation has taken hold. The student will begin to exhibit long-range tranquillity in comparison to the former quick frustration during study activities. When the student can work rather calmly for long periods of time (half an hour or more) with materials that used to bring disruptive reactions, adults will know that remediation has been effective. Then it will be time to take the student to the next step of perceptual development.

Making Referrals. Four out of five dyslexics in the classroom can respond to the techniques suggested in this chapter. Some cannot. Approximately 20% of our handicapped students require specialized remedial therapy away from a group environment. Parents and teachers should call for help when it is indicated. However, classroom teachers must not give up on a child because of the convenience of having him or her placed elsewhere.

Unfortunately, only a handful of clinics and other institutions specialize in dyslexia. Many reading clinics do not deal with this disability. In fact, some clinical services deny that such a reading disability exists. A rule of thumb for referral to other agencies might be this:

> So long as the student is making some progress, I will keep up my efforts to cope with his or her problems. When behavior becomes so disruptive that others cannot learn, or when the student becomes so frustrated that he or she cannot continue in a group, then I will refer that student to another agency for special help.

If there is outside help available for seriously dyslexic students, the classroom teacher can make a trustworthy diagnosis by using the checklists in this book. Many communities are forming volunteer helping-hands groups of interested parents, teenagers, and college students to take some pressure off the disabled students in local classrooms. Churches, civic organizations, and senior citizens are potential allies of the classroom teacher, once such volunteer groups are shown that the need exists.

Principles for Overcoming Visual Dyslexia

This book cannot include all of the techniques for overcoming visual dyslexia. Interested parents and teachers must tailor corrective techniques to fit the specific needs of each student. However, there are some helpful guidelines and principles for working with dyslexic students:

Principle 1: Self-fulfilling Prophecy

Much attention has been drawn to the power that an adult's attitudes exert over the success or failure of students. A general principle can be stated: *Students tend to accomplish what the teacher or parent expects them to accomplish.* In other words, students tend to return the feelings and attitudes they sense in their leaders. If the adult expects youngsters to succeed, they generally will do so. Positive teachers who respect their students are usually respected in return. Negative teachers who regard dyslexics as failures with little hope for success find these pupils failing in class, as well as displaying negative, disrespectful attitudes toward adults. Many studies reveal that test scores and achievement are closely tied to the adult's expectations.

The teacher or parent who prophesies that a student will succeed usually sees pupils achieving success. The adult who predicts failure is not disappointed; those students tend to fail, thus fulfilling the teacher's prophecy.

There is certainly more to success and failure than the teacher's or parents' expectations. But the attitude of the adult is a critical factor for dyslexics. Certain adults are not temperamentally suited for working with dyslexics. When this is the case, every effort should be made to give both adult and student a choice. If working with dyslexics is offensive or uncomfortable for an adult, it will be impossible for a warm, accepting relationship to be established. Students with disabilities do not respond positively to uncomfortable or rigid adults. More harm than good comes from forced associations between adults who dread disabled persons and students who are apprehensive toward adults who feel that way. It is essential that parents and teachers have positive expectations concerning the potential abilities of the handicapped students. If not, the time together will trigger frustration, rebellion, anxiety, and failure.

Principle 2: What Does the Student Need?

Unless teaching techniques actually meet the student's needs, valuable time and energy are wasted and no educational growth is achieved. This principle can be expressed in a practical, 3-point guide:

1. What does the student *need?*
2. What would be *nice* for the student to know?
3. What is *irrelevant* at this time?

In correcting dyslexia, answers to these simplified statements are of great importance. If Paul does not know the alphabet, then learning the alphabet is his *need* of the moment. It would be *nice* for him to read 25 books this year. It would be totally *irrelevant* for him to attempt to write book reports. In other words, if the foundation has never been laid, it is foolish to attempt to build the upper floors. If the student needs the foundation, regardless of age or number of years in school, then the foundation is where the instructor must begin.

Because dyslexics have not fit the standard academic mold, they are termed *disabled.* When parents and teachers discover each student's *need,* as differentiated from what would be *nice* and what is *irrelevant,* then a teaching plan can be developed specifying exact skills the student has failed to learn. This practical approach is simple, direct, and nontheoretical. By filling the student's need, the instructor enables him or her to move on to the things it would be nice to know. As needs are fulfilled, what was irrelevant becomes increasingly more relevant. Adults see students working toward higher level skills surprisingly soon, once a solid foundation has been laid.

Principle 3: Relax the Pressure

The dyslexic student has two mortal enemies: a rapid work rate and pressure for quantity. Dyslexics must work slowly as they write and read. There is no way to make the left brain centers speed up the process of translating language symbols that continually rotate, turn upside down, or refuse to stay fixed in the reader's perception. One of the deadliest experiences for the dyslexic is to be threatened by speed in a reading or writing situation. A universal emotion in dyslexics is panic, particularly when they are forced to work under timed limitations. Rigidly timed standardized tests are especially threatening to most dyslexics. The click of a stopwatch or the starting sound of a timing clock spells doom for these handicapped performers. Time penalties are as cruel for dyslexics as being forced to run in a track meet would be for a person with a withered leg. Adults who are unaware of this panic reaction to time pressure can inflict deep emotional anguish in students whose thought patterns are slow in processing symbols.

Pressure for quantity is equally devastating for dyslexic students. When confronted by assignments that demand a large quantity of work within a limited amount of time, dyslexics give up. A major cause of discipline problems in school and at home is that too much output is expected from handicapped students. Dyslexics normally work several times more slowly than people who are not dyslexic. A rule of thumb for the instructor would be to expect dyslexic students to work three times slower than students without handicaps. This means that if students who are not dyslexic can write 20 sentences in half an hour, dyslexic students would generally do well to complete five or six sentences in the same length of time. If most students in the class can handle five pages of silent reading during a study period, the dyslexic reader would do well to cover one page without help.

When adults allow for these very real limitations in work rate, dyslexics are usually willing to do their best. When handicapped students realize they are being dealt with according to their needs, they tend to respond positively. If given ample time to complete their work, dyslexic students are often the hardest workers in the class. If the purpose of assignments is to strengthen skills, then it does not matter whether conscientious students do 5 or 20 exercises, so long as each class member does his or her best. Teachers set their students up for failure when quantity, rather than quality, becomes the goal.

In dealing with dyslexic learners, parents and classroom teachers may be placed on the defensive by critics who say that it is not fair to "let the dyslexic get out of doing all the work the other students are required to do." However, when adults really believe that every person is entitled to an education according to his or her needs, ways can be found to fill those needs. Relaxing pressure for speed and quantity is a sensible educational objective, especially for students who cannot meet traditional expectations.

Principle 4: Keep It Simple

There is nothing simple about today's school curriculum. Brilliant adults who delight in manipulating complicated theory have designed dozens of advanced programs for elementary and middle schools. Each new textbook adoption startles adults who see difficult concepts being brought into primary and kindergarten education. Pressure is exerted for cramming more and more into the already complex school day of most children. This buildup of high expectations is lethal for dyslexic youngsters who are confused by the bombardment of new information at every turn. Even fun time is so overorganized in many schools that sensitive children dread recess.

Dyslexia involves the inability to sort out sensory impressions satisfactorily. Classroom success is probably not a matter of learning how to react appropriately to the flow of new information. Instead, academic achievement may be the result of learning how *not* to react to the bombardment of stimulus which comes at the student from every side. Dyslexic students usually cannot tune out irrelevant stimulus. They cannot edit the environment to identify what is relevant. When confronted by several stimuli at the same time, dyslexics cannot filter out what is not essential. As a result, mental images are inaccurate, leaving the student unable to cope with all that is expected in today's curriculum.

Dyslexia can be remediated only when outside stimulus factors are carefully controlled. This means that teaching dyslexic students calls for simple, step-by-step routines involving them in only the amount of stimulus they can handle at a given time. For example, when lessons include several concepts, the dyslexic student is overstimulated. Because Paul cannot cope with a variety of expectations at the same time, he fails to comprehend. The result is either neutral (no gain) or negative (loss). However, if dyslexics are guided from one skill to the next at a pace they can handle, eventually they learn to cope with complicated tasks. Parents and teachers who control the amount of stimulus find dyslexic children making surprising progress.

Since the principle of simplicity has always been at the heart of good teaching, curriculum materials are usually programmed to introduce new facts step by step. The problem is not so much with materials or with curriculum goals. The problem is in trying to accomplish too much too quickly. Dyslexics face crushing defeat when they are pressured to hurry through too many skill levels before each level has become habitual or automatic. It is imperative that teachers and parents keep their instruction simple until perceptual foundations are firmly established for handicapped students.

Principle 5: Keep It Structured

No one has estimated the ratio of discoverers to nondiscoverers in our population. Classroom teachers are often confronted by curriculum goals based on the premise that students *will* discover fundamental concepts if they explore enough. Few would deny that certain bright children *can* be led to discover principles and laws if they have sufficient opportunities to explore. However, the fact is that millions of American children are not learning math, spelling, grammar, science, or reading in spite of attractive materials designed to let students explore and discover for themselves.

A cardinal truth regarding learning disability is that *learning new skills must be highly structured.* This principle does not actually contradict modern theories of self-discovery. The fact is that certain students cannot cope with loosely structured situations. Original thinking simply is not possible for many persons until they have experienced specific, structured drill in foundation skills. Dyslexics cannot assemble parts into coherent wholes unless there is a clearly defined model to show them how. Abstract reasoning without visible structure is a major stumbling block for most dyslexics.

Parents and teachers must provide carefully structured, regular teaching routines upon which dyslexic learners can depend. This rules out certain kinds of multiple stimulus activities specified in teachers' manuals and guidebooks. A critical need of disabled learners is for structured guidelines that do not change. Words with multiple meanings, variant spellings of vowel or consonant sounds, open-ended grammar or punctuation rules, and indefinite elements of math, science, and social studies are highly threatening to students who cannot function when things change from lesson to lesson.

3

Overcoming Auditory Dyslexia

Within the dyslexic population is another specific pattern we call auditory dyslexia. This has nothing to do with hearing as such. Most of these strugglers have excellent ability to hear. The problem is that what these students hear is not correctly interpreted by the language processing centers of the left brain. Auditory dyslexics cannot tell differences between certain speech sounds. They continually miss chunks of sound as they listen. They often cannot rhyme words successfully, and they have great difficulty connecting sounds to letters from memory.

One of the most painful experiences for sensitive music teachers and vocal coaches is the monotone student who cannot carry a tune. No matter how much musical drill this person receives, he or she never learns vocal music skills. Fortunately, these tone deaf students can be assigned nonsinging duties when stage productions are prepared. Reading teachers do not have such alternatives for students who are tone deaf to sounds in words. Auditory dyslexia is similar to tone deafness in music. This language disability has little to do with hearing ability. Most auditory dyslexics have keen hearing skills except with phonics. Auditory dyslexia refers to *the inability to hear the separate sounds of spoken language in correct sequence.* Since the student does not hear the building blocks of oral language accurately, he or she cannot connect speech sounds to letters correctly. This disability makes it difficult for students to write their thoughts. Auditory dyslexics usually do not master phonics because they do not make letter/sound connections accurately.

Auditory Dyslexia Syndrome

When diagnosing this disability, teachers and parents must keep in mind that few students master all of the letter/sound relationships of American speech. Most of us have certain areas of phonetic weakness. However, the reading or spelling instructor can learn to identify those students who cannot convert oral language into writing or printed language into correct speech. When trying to read, the auditory dyslexic often does not recognize that written words stand for the spoken words used in daily speech.

A primary characteristic of auditory dyslexia is the inability to hear variations of vowel sounds. Most reading programs emphasize the "long" and "short" sounds of five vowels: *a, e, i, o,* and *u.* Although *w* and *y* are also vowels (called semi-vowels), teachers do not always teach specific sounds for *w* and *y.* Educators have assumed that intelligent students with no speech defects should have no trouble telling the difference between long vowel sounds and short vowel sounds. This is not true with dyslexic students. Auditory dyslexics have great difficulty distinguishing such close words as *big* and *beg* or *cat* and *cot.* For the dyslexic person, subtle distinctions in speech sounds do not exist.

A similar problem is seen when dyslexic students encounter consonant clusters (also called blends and digraphs). Few auditory dyslexics can hear the separate consonant sounds in such clusters as *st, sp, gr,* or *pl.* Dyslexics usually can hear the first consonant letter sound in familiar words. It is frequently impossible for them to hear the second or third sound in clusters like *str, spl,* or *shr.*

It is common for auditory dyslexia to remain undetected during the primary grades, particularly when formal phonics and spelling instruction is postponed until third grade. Nearly all beginner pupils stumble in their first encounters with organized reading and writing instruction. When the whole-word (sight-memory) approach is used in primary grades, teachers can remain unaware that certain pupils are not hearing sounds accurately.

The following sections contain descriptions of symptoms of auditory dyslexia. In addition, a checklist of auditory dyslexia characteristics can be found in Appendix 2.

Confusion with Words: Alike or Different?

One of the earmarks of auditory dyslexia is the student's inability to tell whether words are the same, or whether they are different. Donna is a typical child handicapped by auditory dyslexia. Her teacher has begun to suspect that she does not hear sounds accurately. The teacher used a simple listening test to estimate Donna's auditory perceptual accuracy. Below is a sample of her performance.

> "Donna, listen carefully as I say each set of words. Tell me *Alike* if the two words are exactly the same. Tell me *Different* if the words are not exactly the same."

Pronounced by Teacher	Donna's Responses
"bed–dead"	Different
"dime–time"	Alike
"back–pack"	Alike
"look–look"	Alike
"tam–dam"	Alike
"pane–bane"	Alike
"dill–bill"	Different
"say–say"	Alike
"fat–vat"	Alike
"no–no"	Alike
"hot–what"	Alike
"vetch–fetch"	Alike
"mile–Nile"	Different
"where–hare"	Alike
"got–got"	Alike

A frustrating tendency is sometimes encountered in an activity of this nature. Many dyslexics do not follow instructions well enough to give the kinds of answers the teacher expects. Instead of saying "Alike" or "Different," Donna might say "Yes" or "No," or "Same" and "Not Same." Such behavior should not be regarded as incorrect. The point is to find out whether the student hears sounds accurately, not whether he or she can parrot back stereotyped answers. Much of the conflict in the classroom between dyslexics and teachers is caused when the adult fails to interpret the student's confused signals correctly.

This kind of informal diagnosis reveals some significant deficiencies in Donna's auditory perception. The teacher now has definite guidelines for corrective teaching. This brief activity has revealed Donna's confusion with four sets of similar sound elements: /d/ and /t/, /b/ and /p/, /f/ and /v/, /h/ and /hw/. The teacher will be alert for other areas of faulty perception as she guides Donna's reading and spelling growth. Teachers must be cautious in placing faith in the results of tests like this. Many auditory dyslexics can make perfect scores on this kind of screening instrument. A score on an auditory discrimination test neither establishes nor eliminates a dyslexic condition until other symptoms are also identified.

Mishearing words creates constant problems for auditory dyslexics as they respond to what goes on around them. For example, Donna's teacher kept a record of the misunderstandings that occurred in the girl's listening during one day at school. When the teacher said "leopard," Donna heard *leprosy*. When the teacher said "pity," the girl heard *picky*. When the teacher said "curiosity," Donna heard *cures*. When the teacher said "grief," she heard *grease*. When the teacher said "compare," Donna heard *repair*. When the teacher said "rose," the child heard *roll*. As the teacher discussed "gulf stream," Donna first heard *gull stream*. Later she thought the teacher said *golf stream*. When the teacher said "defends," Donna heard *different*. This kind of record of a student's auditory misperception helps parents and teachers understand much of the conflict that flares up in the student's relationships with others. Every time Donna misunderstood what her teacher said, an argument followed. Because she is bright, Donna wanted to tell what she knew as the words were used by the teacher. Students with this faulty auditory perception are forever darting off on rabbit trails. They go darting away on another topic while everyone else is thinking about what was really said. This creates continual arguments, hurt feelings, misunderstandings, and conflict. It is hard for parents and teachers to realize that Donna is not just being stubborn or difficult. She responds to what she "hears." The message her listening centers receives is not always the same message the speaker said, and this sets her apart when it comes to fitting into her environment.

Confusion with Spelling

Auditory dyslexia is usually the primary cause for habitually poor spelling. Because the student does not hear separate sounds accurately, there is no way to remember how to spell. Traditional spelling instruction is seriously detrimental to auditory dyslexics. When an arbitrary list of unrelated words is assigned on Monday, to be memorized however the student can for Friday's dictation test, the dyslexic student is faced with a frustrating predicament. Intelligent dyslexics frequently devise their own memory systems for remembering spelling patterns ("when" is *h-e-n* with *w* in front; "mother" is *t-h-e* with *mo* in front and *r* at the end). Today's curriculum involving thousands of words presented at an ever faster pace soon produces impossible demands. Few dyslexic individuals are clever enough to figure out memory devices for all the words they must write.

One of the surest symptoms of auditory dyslexia is chronic erasing, crossing out, and marking over (overprinting) to correct written mistakes. A careful observer soon understands why dyslexics struggle through writing activities so nervously. A dyslexic writer usually "thinks out loud" as he or she works, whispering over and over, trying it several ways, erasing, then writing another combination of letters. Students like Donna are never sure they have spelled correctly. Handwriting is a very personal picture of any writer's self. This is especially so for the insecure student who has never been able to please the teacher or parents. Every word committed to paper exposes the dyslexic to probable failure. He or she faces this chronic risk nervously; therefore, the student erases again and again, desperately trying to "luck out" with the correct combinations of letters, hoping to please critics but not really expecting to succeed. Many dyslexics attempt to hide their work as they write, a further indication of their dread of failure.

Certain mistake patterns are seen in the spelling efforts of auditory dyslexics. Four basic patterns of error will be apparent, regardless of the source of the dictation.

Transposed Consonant Elements. Dyslexics habitually change consonant patterns. *Barn* becomes "bran," *play* becomes "paly," and *girl* becomes "gril." The student seldom recognizes these transpositions because of the basic difficulty connecting sounds to letters in the right sequence.

Phonetic Spellings. It is almost impossible for auditory dyslexics to apply phonics rules to spelling. When attempting to write what they hear, dyslexics grope for literal translations. Teachers can spot this tendency if the student's garbled writing is read phonetically. In her attempts to write familiar words, Donna may write "reefews" for *refuse,* or "gard" for *guard.* The old cliché that a child cannot spell *cat* is sometimes true. Many dyslexics write "kat" for *cat* and "cind" for *kind.*

Sound Units Omitted. The most significant indicator of auditory dyslexia in spelling is the habit of leaving out sound units within longer words. This problem is sometimes called *telescoping.* The following examples illustrate this tendency.

Dictated by Teacher	Student's Written Response
remember	rember
extravagance	exstragunce
tuberculosis	toberkulous
candidacy	candiacy
indefinitely	endefinely

Sound Units Added. A further characteristic of auditory dyslexia is the tendency to add unnecessary sound units when writing words. This is also called *perseveration.* This tendency is illustrated below.

Dictated by Teacher	Student's Written Response
duck	dukey
pretty	patting
party	paturing
doll	dalken
blizzard	blizzered
successful	sucessiful
immediate	immediant
intimate	intament
legitimate	lagetiment
zephyr	zesphir

Figure 3.1 shows an effective 15-word dictation test devised by Dr. Ernest Jones. This simple diagnostic instrument allows a teacher or parent to detect auditory dyslexic symptoms quickly. A more complete diagnostic picture for older students can be obtained from dictated word lists that include longer words. Figure 3.2 shows the struggle of a 21-year-old man to write from dictation. He had graduated from high school after spending 13 years trying to master basic literacy skills.

Figure 3.3 and Figure 3.4 show another simple spelling test from the Jordan Written Screening Test (Jordan 1977, 1988b). This is a carefully arranged group of words that are commonly misspelled by dyslexics. Within a few minutes of watching how students encode these words, the teacher can identify dyslexics without causing embarrassment. These examples illustrate how a dictation test reveals confusion with symbols, as well as dyslexic tendencies to reverse, rotate, and transpose letters.

Auditory dyslexia is a major handicap when students try to write essay answers or produce original stories or themes. Dyslexic spelling is frequently associated with dysgraphia (see Chapter 4). It is not difficult to see the symptoms of auditory dyslexia in a student's written work, if parents and teachers analyze handwritten papers carefully.

Figure 3.5 shows an example of dyslexic writing by a bright girl in fourth grade. Her autobiography was brushed aside as the work of a retarded child until her teachers discovered that the girl was dyslexic, not retarded. This example illustrates a combination of auditory dyslexia (faulty letter/sound connecting) and dysgraphia (inability to

dig	deg	dig	dit
for	for	for	for
pig	pig	pig	pig
barn	brne	brnu	lar
say	see	Say	sand
pretty	pette	prite	pelling
kind	cice	cind	kin
brown	bown	brond	brown
party	prtte	prtey	patting
on	on	on	no
duck	Diik	dukey	duck
bear	Bare	beru	bru
doll	Ball	dill	dalkin
ate	ate	ate	eat
goes	gose	gos	gose

Figure 3.1. A dictation test. These are classic auditory spelling patterns as three students tried to write the 15 words from dictation.

write legibly). Below the writing sample is a typed "translation" to reveal the auditory dyslexic spelling flaws more clearly.

Figure 3.6 shows extremely dyslexic writing by a college student who was 20 years old. She was enrolled as a special education major, hoping to become certified to teach children with learning disabilities. A sympathetic professor recognized this student's dyslexic patterns

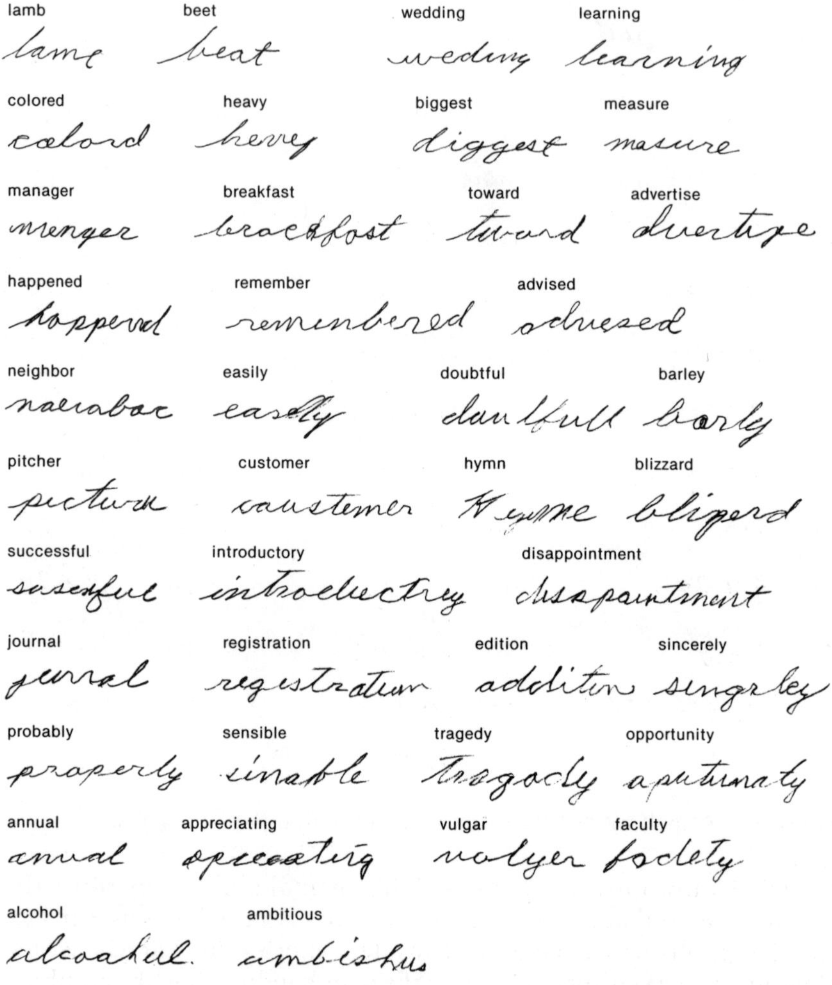

lamb beet wedding learning

colored heavy biggest measure

manager breakfast toward advertise

happened remember advised

neighbor easily doubtful barley

pitcher customer hymn blizzard

successful introductory disappointment

journal registration edition sincerely

probably sensible tragedy opportunity

annual appreciating vulgar faculty

alcohol ambitious

Figure 3.2. A dictation test administered to a 21-year-old man. The student required more than 30 minutes to write these words. He had to whisper over and over with frequent erasing. He was exhausted when he finished this dictated spelling test.

---

and began working with her one-to-one. She developed word processor skills that allowed her to bypass her dyslexic writing problems.

No one knows how many intelligent, creative students have been written off as academic failures because adults have not known how to identify dyslexia. Figure 3.7 shows part of an original story Larry wrote when he was 15 years old. A poorly administered intelligence test had labeled him Borderline Retarded with IQ 72. When his

Word	Response	Word	Response	Word	Response
dig	DEG	pig	piG	big	BiG
ate	ATE	rode	roD	goes	GOeS
play	plAgy	please	pLeS	toes	ToeS
duck	DOuCK	buck	Bouke	truck	TrKe
party	pArty	pretty	prtey	try	Try
brown	Brown	born	BerN	for	For
barn	BArN	brand	Brdne	from	From
girl	GrALe	bird	BreDy	stop	STOP
saw	SAW	was	WAS	post	POST
kind	KinDe	king	KinG	slat	sLATe
city	City	cent	SenT	salt	SLot
this	these	think	thAnK	how	haw
on	ON	no	no	who	ho

Figure 3.3. A spelling test from the Jordan Written Screening Test.

dyslexic handicaps were diagnosed, his mental ability was correctly measured as well above average. He sent five original manuscripts to a major publisher of paperback mystery stories. To Larry's astonishment, an alert editor deciphered the poor handwriting (dysgraphia) and discovered the story lines that Larry had created. The editor returned the manuscripts with a lengthy critique, advising the boy what to do to improve his stories. He encouraged Larry to keep sending story ideas, pointing out that the publisher was interested in purchasing fresh story material. With this unique incentive, Larry became interested in school achievement for the first time in his life. He quickly developed good writing ability with a word processor. It is a sobering thought that this bright young man had been labeled hopeless by teachers who had not recognized the potential behind his disabilities.

Confusion with Rhyming Elements. An easily detected characteristic of auditory dyslexia is difficulty with rhyme. As a standard

Word	Written	Word	Written	Word	Written
dig	dig	pig	pige	big	big
ate	ate	rode	rod	goes	gos
play	gla	please	ples	toes	toce
duck	dog	buck	bog	track	troc
party	prte	pretty	pretey	try	tria
brown	bron	born	brne	for	fore
barn	brna	brand	brand	from	fom
girl	grle	bird	brd	stop	stop
saw	sou	was	wos	post	post
kind	kind	king	ben	slat	slat
city	cite	cent	sint	salt	solt
this	thes	think	thac	how	haw
on	on	no	no	who	hoh

Figure 3.4. A spelling test. This dyslexic student learned cursive writing, which is unusual for someone with this much struggle to encode. Notice that most of the circular letters are made with backward strokes.

practice in elementary reading instruction, most teachers dwell on rhyming words to reinforce pupil awareness of sounds in words. Students handicapped by auditory dyslexia have great difficulty hearing likenesses and differences in words. Awkwardness in hearing or saying rhymes is a major symptom of this disability.

Educators probably make too great an issue of faulty rhyming ability. Aside from providing a convenient vehicle for phonics drills, rhyming skill is actually of little practical importance, so far as overall reading maturity is concerned. The ability to rhyme does help many children master writing and spelling. It is unfortunate that children with poor rhyming skill are often penalized. Adults should remember that many students who do oral rhyming activities well cannot do so in writing. To be sure of the extent of the disability, the teacher must use both oral and written activities.

An example of this informal procedure is to ask the student to name all the words he or she can rhyme with *car*. A student with

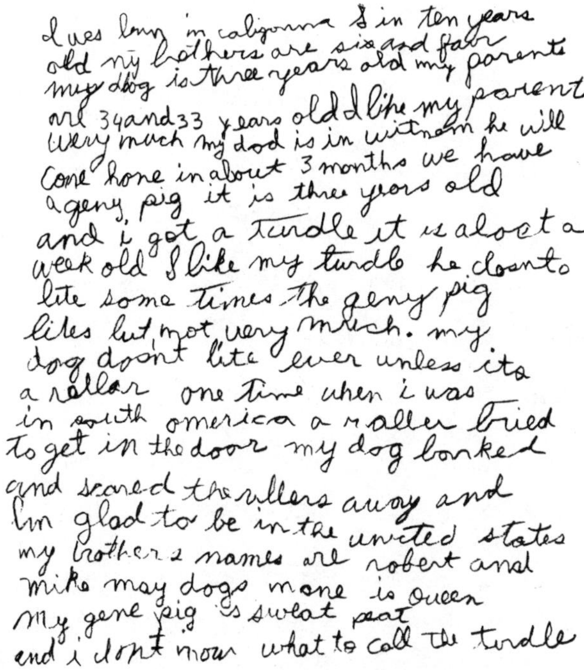
I wes born in caligorrna S in ten years
old my brothers are six and four
my dog is three years old my parents
are 34and33 years old I like my parents
wery much my dad is in witnam he will
come home in about 3 months we have
a geny pig it is three years old
and i got a turdle it is aloot a
week old S like my turdle he doesnt
lite some times the geny pig
lites but mot very much. my
dog doesnt lite ever unless its
a rollar one time when i was
in south omerica a roller tried
to get in the door my dog barked
and scared the rillers away and
Im glad to be in the united states
my brothers names are robert and
mike may dogs mone is Queen
my gene pig is swlat peat
and i dont now what to call the turdle

I was born in califarna (California) S (I) in (am) ten years old my brothers are six and four my dog is three years old my parents are 34 and 33 years old I like my parents wery (very) much my dad is in watnam (Vietnam) he will come home in about 3 months we have a geny (Guinea) pig it is three years old and i got a turdle (turtle) it is aloud (about) a week old S (I) like my turdle he dosnt (doesn't) lite (bite) some times the geny pig lites (bites) but mot (not) very much. my dog dosn't bite ever unless its a rolber (robber). one tine (time) vhen (when) i was in south america a ruller (robber) tried to get in the door my dog barked and scared the rillers (robbers) away and Im (I'm) glad to be in the united states, my brothers names are robert and Mike may (my) dogs (dog's) name is Oueen (Queen) my gene pig is sweat peat (Sweet Pete) and i dont now (know) what to call the turdle.

Figure 3.5. A writing sample produced by a 9-year-old girl. Later she developed excellent writing skills with a word processor that helped her find misspelled words.

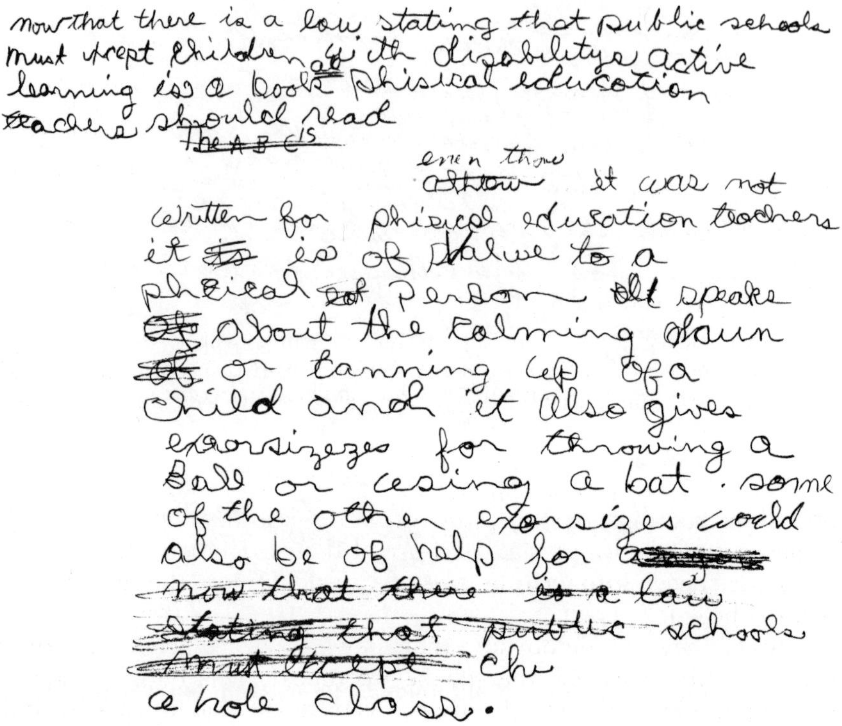

now that there is a law stating that public schools
must accept children with disabilitys active
learning is a book phisical education
teachers should read
~~The ABC's~~

even though ~~althow~~ it was not
written for phisical education teachers
it ~~is~~ is of value to a
phisical ~~ed~~ person it speaks
~~of~~ about the calming down
~~of~~ or tanning up of a
child and it also gives
exorsizezes for throwing a
ball or using a bat. some
of the other exorsizes would
also be of help for ~~[illegible]~~
~~now that there is a law~~
~~stating that public schools~~
~~must accept~~ chi
a hole class.

Figure 3.6. A sample of dyslexic writing. This 20-year-old student finally earned a special education teaching certificate and became an excellent teacher with learning disabled youngsters.

normal perception should respond quickly with such words as *jar, far, star, bar.* If the student needs a lot of time to ponder through each word before saying it, he or she may be handicapped by auditory dyslexia. This will be particularly evident if the student names nonsense words, such as *dar, sar, nar, har, zar.* Dyslexics often name words that begin alike but do not rhyme, such as *car, care, core, cure.* If the student cannot match printed rhyming words, or if he or she cannot write familiar rhyming words by substituting beginning consonants, the teacher can be reasonably sure that an auditory dyslexic condition exists.

Need for Speaker to Repeat. An especially irritating characteristic for many teachers is the dyslexic's need for repetition. Auditory dyslexic students are insecure, especially in the classroom. They often feel very ill-at-ease in school because they cannot make letter/sound connections accurately. When writing from dictation or following a series

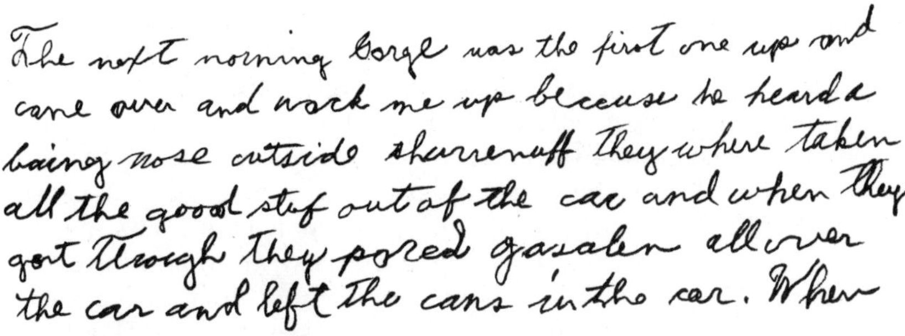

The next morning Gorge was the first one up and
came over and wock me up because he heard a
baing nose outside sharrenuff they where taken
all the good stuf out of the car and when they
got though they pored gasalen all over
the car and left the cans in the car. When

Figure 3.7. Notice the extremely small handwriting of this dyslexic student. Occasionally a severely dyslexic person develops tiny writing partly to hide mistakes in spelling. Larry filled several notebooks with this kind of creative story writing.

of oral instructions, dyslexic students simply cannot cope with a sustained flow of oral material. Because of their extremely slow rate in changing speech into writing, auditory dyslexics lose the sequence of what is heard.

Since they are seldom sure that they have heard accurately, dyslexics continuously ask the speaker to repeat. This habit produces friction in many learning situations. As dyslexic students fall behind the group, they tend to become disruptive. Discipline problems often stem from the subtle, invisible presence of tone-deaf listening. It is not unusual for dyslexics to be shunned by their peers who are annoyed by their "weird" behavior and disruptive habits. Struggling to hold their social position creates friction, which results in a lot of conflict with adult authority. What begins as a dyslexic flaw often leads to social problems and public embarrassment. Yet little of this poor behavior is deliberate on the part of dyslexics.

Subvocalizing During Silent Reading. A common image of classroom teachers is snapping of fingers followed by "Shhhhhhhh!" For many years students have been taught that making vocal sounds during silent reading time is forbidden. Perhaps the practice of forbidding subvocalization does improve learning for certain students, although it is probably more beneficial to the teacher's frazzled nerves than to growth in reading skills. The truth is that dyslexic students *must* subvocalize if they are to succeed in translating writing into meaningful thought. Because of the underlying problem in connecting sounds to letters, dyslexic readers must use several brain pathways to verify their impressions. A person with no impairment can learn to read just by seeing the page. A dyslexic student cannot.

This frustrating need to reinforce seeing with saying, along with touching words with a finger, should not upset parents or teachers. It is not difficult to let dyslexic students use their unorthodox ways if the teacher is aware of the problem. The important thing is that dyslexics must respond to reading in a variety of ways to check their impressions for accuracy. When the teacher snaps her fingers and hisses "Shhhhhhhh!" she is cutting off an essential learning channel for auditory dyslexics. The result is increased frustration and failure.

This need to reinforce seeing with voice and touch also appears when auditory dyslexics are doing written assignments. These students need to whisper during spelling tests and while writing stories or essays. If dyslexics are allowed to cross-check their impressions by speaking as they write, they can learn to correct many mistakes and spelling. If they are allowed to touch their words and whisper, they can learn to read much better.

Difficulty Blending Parts into Word Wholes. In Chapter 1 an example was given of Donna's attempt to read aloud from a science text. The heart of her reading handicap is faulty blending. This leaves her unable to cope with one of the major skills of accurate word analysis. The entire auditory dyslexic syndrome seems to focus upon Donna's problems in "sounding out" words as she reads. For example, a familiar word like *bug* can become a major hurdle for the dyslexic reader. Laboriously Donna breaks the word apart: "buh-uh-guh." As this effort illustrates, she has never learned the right way to say the consonants *b* and *g*. When she feels somewhat confident that she has the separate sounds in mind, Donna takes the plunge: "blug." Again she has failed. *Yellow* comes out "yelelow," and *bridge* turns into "burge." Students like Donna quickly grow defensive and insecure when forced to expose themselves to such public failure.

Traditional instruction in phonics which emphasizes blending is usually beyond the comprehension of auditory dyslexics. It is possible for students like Donna to achieve success in simple word analysis after a lot of drill and memorization of key word patterns. This technique, called *overteaching,* saturates the student with intensive, highly structured practice with regular words until an automatic response occurs. Students like Donna seldom develop true understanding of blending and word analysis, although they often can learn to read.

Garbled Pronunciation. Closely associated with the inability to blend is an embarrassing problem of garbled pronunciation. Auditory dyslexics find themselves the object of much laughter and teasing because of scrambled speech. Parents and teachers can identify this aspect of dyslexia by devising lists of words for the student to repeat. This scrambled speech is also called *echolalia*.

Normal Pronunciation	**Auditory Dyslexic Speech**
aluminum	alunimum
vinegar	vigenar
animals	aminals
olive	olly
baskets	baksets
streamline	steamline
spaghetti	pasghetti

Teachers and students can have fun with pronunciation games which reveal echolalia in which sound units are scrambled within words. For example, the teacher might have the class do a "Tongue Twister Race," keeping a diagnostic record of garbled speech tendencies of certain students. The emphasis must be upon fun with no one feeling shame because of a twisted tongue. Below are some good word combinations for this informal diagnosis:

apples in cinnamon
alum in vinegar
baskets of olives
she sells sea shells on the seashore
aluminum animals
Mama's spaghetti
transcontinental train

Older students enjoy such twisters as these:

political candidacy
musketry maneuvers
blueberry strudel
a crow flew over the river with a lump of raw liver
six long, slim, sleek, slick, slender saplings

Confusion with Dictionary Symbols. As would be expected, auditory dyslexia makes traditional dictionary usage quite difficult for handicapped students. To expect dyslexics to interpret phonetic respellings, accent markings, and pronunciation guides is usually unrealistic. Intelligent, highly motivated students with dyslexic tendencies do manage to cope with the various codes found in reference materials. However, most dyslexic children cannot comprehend the variety of symbol systems they see in recent dictionaries. This problem is further complicated by the use of schwa symbols showing vowel sounds in unaccented syllables. Dyslexic students can benefit from studies in word origins, multiple meanings, and syllable division, but to arrive at correct word pronunciation from dictionary keys is frequently impossible.

Learning Activities for Auditory Dyslexia

It is imperative that dyslexic students have highly structured, well-organized learning procedures that do not change from day to day. Equally important is keeping materials, tools, reference books, and so forth in the same place in the classroom. Oral instructions, written instructions, and placement of materials must be consistent. Once dyslexic students learn where things are, they depend on those things being in the same places day after day. Keeping the learning environment well organized without surprise changes is essential. If the classroom arrangement must be changed, dyslexic students must relearn the landmarks before they feel comfortable again. The following guidelines will help to establish a well-organized learning environment in which dyslexic students can learn comfortably.

Organizing the Classroom

Auditory dyslexics do not respond to the usual practice of presenting a rule, then practicing that rule with words that follow the rule. Instead, dyslexics must begin with structured experience. At a later time they may understand the rule, although many dyslexics never fully comprehend the rules. They can gain a level of functional performance without being able to tell why or how they carry out the rule. Since independent literacy is the goal of education, this functional level must be considered good enough.

If one is dyslexic, all of the senses must be involved in becoming a functional reader or speller. This immediately poses problems for classroom management. The teacher's dilemma is to provide for the different learning styles she finds among her pupils. This can be accomplished if the teacher keeps her sense of humor, is not too rigid, and remembers that students are human beings with exactly the same feelings an adult has experienced in the toughest high school or college course he or she ever took. If it had not been for mercies extended by sympathetic professors, many excellent classroom teachers would never have gained professional certification.

There are literally thousands of ideas in professional publications for teaching reading, writing, and spelling skills to perceptually handicapped children. The teacher of dyslexics must keep in mind the cardinal principles for these handicapped children: simplicity, repetition, and step-by-step progression into higher-level skill areas. Almost any teaching technique can be made to fit the needs of dyslexics if the pace is kept slow enough and the drill work simple and thorough.

Before dyslexics begin to become functional with letter/sound connections, they must have a great deal of experience with stable word patterns that follow the rules the teacher hopes to teach. The most practical source of words is the daily vocabulary of the students. It is a disturbing fact, yet one educators cannot deny, that many dyslexics will not finish school. Therefore, they need to master the basic skills of functional literacy if they are to manage their own affairs when formal schooling is over.

Establishing a Utility Corner. Basal readers, spelling manuals, language handbooks, and arithmetic and social studies textbooks are virtually meaningless to most dyslexic children. This is not to criticize the materials or their authors. The point is that textbooks designed for the average, middle-achieving student are not geared for the extremely slow reaction time of the dyslexic. Because of their different styles of learning, Paul's and Donna's literacy skills must be geared to their immediate daily environment. Although they are capable of imagination, dyslexic students are usually Number Three (physical) learners or Number Two learners who must see it/say it/hear it (see Principle 3 later in this chapter for a definition of learner types). This being true, the dyslexic's quest for independent reading, spelling, writing, and arithmetic skills must take a different course. The most direct route is through the experiences these students encounter every day, although this detour away from textbooks traumatizes many parents and teachers.

The most effective classroom device for enlisting the interest and cooperation of auditory dyslexics is a utility corner, or whatever the teacher and students want to call it. This technique is as effective with adolescents and adults as it is with kindergartners. The need is to create a permanent place in the classroom where utility words are displayed. Two or three shelves of common grocery items are needed, displaying food labels that everyone should know how to read and spell. Included are the prices, needed to teach simple money figuring. In addition to the grocery shelves are other utility items, such as clothing, utensils, tools, sports and recreation equipment, parts for motor bikes or cars, items for good grooming, common medical supplies, and whatever else is appropriate to the interests and lifestyles of the students involved.

In addition to these tangible objects, other utility word sources should be provided: sections of the daily newspaper; a Bible for religiously oriented students; mail order catalogs; phone and city directories; maps of city and state; travel guidebooks from major oil companies. For older students there should be samples of checkbooks and budget planning materials; cookbooks; income tax forms; applications for fishing, hunting, and driver's licenses; manuals outlining local hunting, fishing, and motor vehicle regulations; and reproductions of traffic signs. There should be a browsing table for popular magazines the students bring to exchange, as well as comic books and paperbacks they have enjoyed. There should be a guide for television shows and reviews of movies, as well as current magazines on easy reading levels.

All of this is not for entertainment, and it need not occupy much space. The utility corner is absolutely practical, as well as essential for treating dyslexia in the classroom. The packages and other materials provide immediate visual cues through colors, shapes, word forms, and unique patterns. These cues trigger quick recall of important information for students with faulty retrieval. Here the teacher finds a wealth of simple, practical language materials for teaching literacy, which is the primary social need of dyslexics. Of course, it would be nice if the students could spend time with their textbooks. But until they can function in the marketplace, textbooks are largely irrelevant.

Even primary children need to master a basic reading, writing, and spelling vocabulary of utility terms. Perhaps every teacher should live as dyslexics live for a while, not knowing which door leads to the right restroom, not knowing how to find specific streets or house numbers, not being able to order a meal from a menu, not knowing how to deposit money in a bank or how to make or follow a shopping list, and not being able to write the simplest kind of letter. The utility corner opens up many new doors into face-saving independence, as well as providing the teacher with ready-made sources of instructional activities.

Every important phonics rule can be taught from the utility corner. For example, the grocery shelves are loaded with word families: the *-am* family (*ham, jam, Pam, Spam, yam*). Variant spelling patterns are easily illustrated: *steak, cake, weight.* Homonyms are evident, particularly in traffic terminology: *right–write, wait–weight, road–rode.* Also at the teacher's fingertips are words to illustrate rules about dividing words into syllables:

1. Dividing between consonants that are alike (double consonants)
   but/ter dol/lar car/rot ham/mer pep/per cab/bage

2. Dividing between consonants that are not alike
   tur/key sil/ver quar/ter Hon/da Mus/tang
3. Dividing after the vowel in open syllables
   ba/con rhu/barb pe/can to/ma/to Che/velle
4. Dividing between speaking vowel units
   Bu/ick Toy/o/ta su/et O/hi/o ra/di/o
5. Compound words
   straw/berry pine/apple police/man
   ice cream hot dog post office

The utility corner is a prime source of creative writing ideas, if the quantity of writing is kept small. With the many sensory cues from pictures, packages, colors, shapes, and flavors, there is a wealth of quick stimulus material. Dyslexic students find it much easier to write acceptably when this kind of cue library is at hand. It is personal because they have helped assemble the items in the utility corner. It is familiar because of the interaction and discussions triggered by the materials. The principal value is that this corner is theirs. It is not something the teacher has dictated from an impersonal, overwhelming textbook. With this sort of local authority on hand, the teacher is now prepared to hold her dyslexic students accountable for reasonable quotas of achievement, just as she holds other students accountable for material from their textbooks. In other words, now that materials have been accumulated to meet individual needs, it is time for everyone in the class to get to work.

Dyslexics should not be pampered any more than their peers. Once the teacher has provided learning sources within the skill ranges of her learners, dyslexic students can be held accountable for this material. If the others are expected to master 20 spelling words each week from a regular grade level text, the utility corner students can meet a similar expectation, scaled down to their levels of literacy. Occasionally the teacher will have a handicapped student who cannot cope with the same quantity of output as other dyslexics. His or her productive rate should be determined, then the student should be held accountable for what can be done at his or her own pace. Since some dyslexics work as much as five times slower than others, productivity should be geared to the student's ability to maintain a steady work rate.

The utility corner is only a starting place. If Paul and Donna should not finish their formal education, at least they can shop for groceries and fill out a job application form. The hope is that by starting with a practical base in the utility corner, each dyslexic will eventually transfer his or her literacy skills to textbook materials. It is essential, however, that this transfer not be forced. As the foundations for literacy are laid, most dyslexics will want to move on to more sophisticated reading, writing, and spelling attainment. Influence of peers is largely responsible for this kind of maturity. There is a reason why dyslexics in traditional classroom settings show so little interest in becoming involved in textbook and library reading. It is because such activities have been forced by anxious adults before the students could handle these expectations with any comfort or pleasure. When a boy finds himself comprehending used car ads, or when a girl is able to understand a recipe from the back of a sugar package, then each is approaching the next step of independent reading, that of interpreting similar materials in book form. But this transition is extremely sensitive. When adults push too hard too soon for more mature reading behaviors, dyslexics revert to their old habits of avoidance and rebellion. The utility corner is largely a rest stop along the way. The purpose is to build self-confidence on a practical, day-to-day basis in the area in which these students really live. When they are comfortable, most of them will volunteer to leave the utility corner for more abstract areas of education.

Creating an Interaction Center. Overcoming auditory dyslexia in the classroom depends upon one vital element: *interaction.* If this factor is missing from the dyslexic's learning environment, then very little formal skill development will occur. The styles of learning described later in this chapter (see Principle 3) suggest that several forms of interaction may be needed within a classroom (Jordan, 1988b). No one can expect a teacher working alone with many students to satisfy all the needs of her learners. The utility corner is one way to stimulate certain learning styles so the student can start producing. Establishing an interaction center is another.

Interaction involves physical movement, listening, and speaking. Auditory dyslexics must experience all three aspects of interaction in order to integrate the elements of reading, writing, and spelling. In other words, they need to feel it, hold it, manipulate it, hear it, say it, and act it out, if necessary. This usually cannot occur at the reading circle or when the dyslexic student is confined to his or her seat.

The teacher's first problem with interaction is keeping the noise level under control. Number One learners (who learn better in silence) are greatly irritated and frustrated by movement and sounds elsewhere in the room. If the interaction center has some kind of acoustical control, such as a few square yards of thick carpet, the sounds of interchange can be tolerated within the classroom.

It is usually possible to create an interaction center within a regular classroom, if only for a few minutes at a time. Ideally, the center should be partially screened by bookshelves or portable partitions. The point is to separate Number One learners from Number Two's and Three's (see Principle 3 at end of this chapter). If the teacher counsels students about accepting each other's needs, this arrangement usually proves satisfactory. It will not be perfect, but few teachers are accustomed to perfect conditions.

The interaction center is primarily for the purpose of oral and kinesthetic interchange. For 10 or 15 minutes each day, the teacher meets those learners who need body involvement for comprehension. This is the place to try Dr. Duggin's kinesthetic techniques for comprehending vowel qualities. This is also the place to let dyslexics use their bodies in role playing as they try to associate meaning with symbols: *hop* as you say each letter to learn *h-o-p*; *skip* four times to learn *s-k-i-p*; *roll over* four times while saying *o-v-e-r*. When auditory dyslexic children are involved in this kind of body learning, an amazing growth in literacy often occurs. Once the combined learning channels have imprinted the concept in the learner's memory, it is usually there to stay. The interaction center can accomplish more in a month than a quiet, passive remedial reading class can produce in a year in most cases of auditory dyslexia.

A remarkable discovery has been made by a number of teachers who have provided interaction centers in their classrooms. A sturdy rocking chair can become an avenue of learning, particularly for overly active students. Many dyslexics feel themselves becoming more and more tense as the school day wears on. In fact, these hypertensive students talk in terms of feeling like "I'm about to explode." There is no provision made in most classrooms for releasing this pent-up energy without creating a disruptive situation which distracts others. The rocking chair is an ideal lightning rod for discharging potentially destructive friction in struggling learners. An agreement is usually made that, when no one else is using the rocker, a student like Paul who finds himself tense may take his book to the interaction center. There he may rock and read for a few minutes until he feels like returning to his seat. If the rocker is placed on carpeting there is almost no noise to disturb others at work. In many classrooms the rocking chair has helped save the sanity of hypertensive learners and harassed teachers. The by-products are increased learning, decreased disruptive behavior, and remarkably improved achievement levels of those who need to rock away inner frustrations of the moment.

An interaction center creates a new possibility for both teacher and learner. For the first time, alternate styles of behavior can be tolerated. This means that dyslexics who generate friction when they rub their associates the wrong way now have an acceptable way to disperse their tension. Ordinarily the teacher either bottles up his or her irritations or immediately strikes out at the offending student. If the teacher holds back his or her true feelings, genuine hostility develops toward the student. In turn, the student senses the teacher's attitudes and begins to resent and fear the teacher's authority. Sooner or later their relationship disintegrates into a confrontation which not only further deteriorates their mutual feelings but also upsets other students and adults involved. This is the universal dilemma of how to coexist with disabled learners in the classroom. In the mainstream classroom where there are no alternatives, there is virtually no joy, and usually not much learning for the struggling learner.

Although it is difficult to provide well-stocked utility corners and interaction centers within already crowded classrooms, the effort to do so pays good dividends. Merely demonstrating to disabled students that their needs are being considered is sometimes enough to create a positive working relationship between them and the teacher. The major problems of teaching and learning may persist, but efforts to provide alternatives almost always result in academic progress, even when the teacher cannot provide for all the needs in the room. Overcoming dyslexia begins with removal of inner barriers within the attitudes and expectations of adults and learners. The teacher need not be concerned so much with the facilities at hand as with new outlets to drain off the frustrations of dyslexia in the classroom.

Making Letter/Sound Connections Through Multisensory Techniques

The point has been made that overcoming auditory dyslexia requires a multisensory approach involving all the senses that can be brought together in the learning process. The four most basic learning channels are sight, sound, speech, and touch. When these sensory pathways are integrated, auditory dyslexics begin to comprehend what reading, spelling, writing, and math computation are all about. Glass Analysis, Touch Math, the *Type-Write Program,* and D'Nealian handwriting are excellent commercial products for this kind of remediation.

Identifying Sound Chunks in Spoken Words. Some teachers think only of consonants and vowels when reference is made to sounds within spoken words. These elements of language instruction are not the beginning points for auditory dyslexics. Instead, beginning emphasis must be placed upon hearing syllable chunks and whole words. If sight, sound, speech, and touch can be brought together in this experience, it is possible to bypass tone deafness to word elements.

Hundreds of activities for teaching dyslexics how to identify sound chunks can be found in professional literature, but the emphasis is the same. The child must connect how the word looks to how it sounds. This is best done by incorporating muscle reactions through the hands, feet, mouth, or whole body. Even for dyslexic adults the process is the same; see it, say it, hear it, feel it, and if necessary, act it out. An integrated variety of sensory impressions must be poured into the learning activity.

Stepping Off the Syllables. For many years younger children have been drilled in word perception through games. These are often accompanied by music, as in simple kindergarten games in which body movements keep time with chanted lyrics. Skipping rope while chanting a rhyme is a playground activity illustrating this principle. But because there are no visual patterns of the words or syllables being chanted, such games seldom lead dyslexic children to make letter/sound connections.

Beginner students are frequently taught by placing letters or words on the floor. Then the children hop, skip, or jump from letter to letter (or word to word) while singing a song or chanting a rhyme. This simple activity is quite effective in memorizing alphabet sequence or a basic sight-memory vocabulary. For older dyslexics who are extremely self-conscious, less obvious routines are needed in the classroom.

Tapping Out the Syllables. Probably the most effective classroom techniques for teaching students to identify chunks in words are arm tapping or chin bumping. First the printed word is displayed, along with pictures and brief explanations of its meaning. The students repeat the word as the teacher monitors to be sure everyone is understanding the pronunciation correctly. Then, if the word has two or more chunks, the group practices tapping out the syllables, keeping time with their own pronunciations. For some reason, clapping the hands is not always effective with dyslexics. Tapping, as described below, seems more universally effective than clapping.

For example, *turkey* is broken into two sound chunks. Care is taken not to cause the student to think of the chunks as two words. A picture is displayed along with the word which is printed on a flash card. The teacher separates the syllable chunks visually by cutting the word, allowing the syllable chunks to be moved apart, then back together. This illustrates how the chunks go together to make the whole word. Then the students use the first two fingers of the writing hand to tap the opposite forearm (left-handed pupils would tap with their left hands). Sometimes a very light tap is enough. Occasionally a dyslexic child will react only to a sharp slapping of fingers against forearm. The important thing is for the student to get a simultaneous, four-part sensation all at once with vision, sound, speech, and touch coming together at the same time.

It is important that the teacher move the syllable cards in time to the oral pronunciation of each syllable. The dyslexic students must see the syllable chunks actually blending together to form the word at the same moment they feel their fingers tap their arms. All of this occurs as the voice says the rhythm of the syllables. The teacher will be aware of how much of this drill each word requires. Simple words like *turkey* will require minimal drill. More complicated words like *unconscious* call for considerably more drill involving sight, sound, speech, and movement.

Counting Chin Bumps. Another way to find the chunks in a word is chin bumping, used many years ago to teach syllable division. Instead of tapping fingers against the forearm, the student says the word slowly, feeling the drop of the chin as he or she says each syllable. This often calls for exaggerated speech so the chin movement will be obvious. This simple technique of marking oral chunks is so reliable, in fact, that it can be used with surprising accuracy. In applying readability formulas to establish the difficulty levels of library materials, researchers often count their chin bumps rather than rely on visual syllable counts. The disadvantage is that chin bump syllables do not always match dictionary syllable division. Dictionary usage is based more upon technical language rules than upon the way words are actually said. Chin bumping and arm tapping are tried-and-true classroom techniques for integrating sight, sound, speech, and body movements to overcome dyslexic handicaps in perceiving letter/sound connections.

An essential outcome of finger tapping or chin bumping is the ability to track through the sequence of sounds accurately. As described in Chapter 1 and earlier in this chapter, auditory dyslexics tend to garble the pronunciation of many common words. This involves the failure to follow the sequence of sound chunks through the spoken word. Tapping out syllables provides excellent corrective training for faulty sequence. For example, if Donna fails to hear middle syllables, she should tap or count her chin bumps while the teacher moves the syllable cards together. If she fails to hear or say a syllable chunk accurately, the teacher does not move the visual cue card. Thus Donna has a visual reminder of her speaking/listening deficiency. She is also confronted by a structured, tangible guideline for correcting this perceptual error.

Some dyslexics must stay with this kind of basic perceptual practice for many months. Others quickly learn to transfer these chunking skills to whatever materials they encounter in reading. It is important that teachers *not* mix traditional phonics with syllable chunking. It is essential that auditory dyslexics approach word analysis from the whole word (or whole syllable) angle first. Once they have comprehended how syllables go together to make up whole words, then they can begin to break syllable chunks into individual vowel or consonant sounds.

Using the Typewriter or Word Processor and Tape Recorder. The value of the typewriter and word processor in the classroom has only recently been recognized by educators. Because of the cost of new machines, most teachers have simply put out of their minds the possibility of having a keyboard unit in the classroom. Traditional school emphasis upon penmanship for everyone has further obscured the potential that typewriters and word processors hold for remediation of dyslexia.

As discussed in chapters 1 and 4, dysgraphic students are especially handicapped by their inability to cope with all of the handwriting expectations. Auditory dyslexia poses a similar threat for those who cannot recall word patterns correctly. When disabled students are taught how to write with a keyboard, a new world of possibilities emerges.

As our culture approaches the 21st century, there is less and less need for mastery of traditional penmanship. Electronic firms that specialize in business machines are predicting that doing jobs by handwriting may become obsolete in the foreseeable future. With new families of electronic devices already on the market, dysgraphic and dyslexic persons will be able to enter professions that now require spelling, handwriting, and composition skills. In an era of voice recorders and automatic typing machines, which offer a variety of options for encoding messages and retrieving information, the classroom should at least introduce children to these alternative forms of writing.

Every classroom needs at least one keyboard system, along with a tape recorder equipped with earphones for privacy. A typewriter need not be new or expensive. In fact, it is better to have an old typewriter that cannot be damaged easily. Extremely slow work rate will force most dyslexic students to "hunt and peck" when typing out words until they have been trained with the *Type-Write Program* or a similar keyboard approach. The emphasis is never upon typing speed, but rather upon encoding letters in correct sequence to spell out words accurately.

The typewriter or word processor is not intended to replace all penmanship. The value of keyboard writing with dyslexics is to give physical reinforcement of sight and sound patterns in words. When integrated with a tape recorder, the keyboard can be a valuable adjunct to the utility corner and interaction center.

The keyboard–tape recorder routine is quite simple. The point of this activity is to provide an integrated experience with sight, sound, speech, and touch. The words can be taken from any source, preferably from the student's own vocabulary needs. The routine is for the dyslexic to study a word on a card, pronouncing the word into the microphone of the tape recorder. The student spells the word aloud into the recorder. Then the word is typed immediately from memory. Next the student reads into the microphone the way the word was typed. Then the student selects another word card and repeats this process. After spelling out five words, the student runs the tape back to the starting position and reviews what was typed and spoken into the recorder. The student continues this routine, five words in each work segment, until all the words in the card set have been done.

Almost immediately dyslexics using the keyboard become aware of the sequence of letters within the words being typed and recorded. Any reversal or rotation tendencies will quickly become apparent. The teacher may overhear a student like Paul muttering as he hunts and pecks away behind his earphones: "Where's the b? Uh, oh! I got it upside down again. Now, where's o? a-b-o-v-e. Above!" This stream of chatter is almost exactly the thought pattern a dyslexic student experiences with every school assignment. Listening to a dyslexic work his or her way through an exercise with the keyboard and recorder will reveal much about dyslexic confusion with symbols.

Recruiting Teacher Aides

The Bible records a remarkable lesson in how a frustrated, overworked leader solved a major problem of group management. Moses tried to handle all the details, giving personal attention to the needs of a million people. Jethro, observing his son-in-law struggling to do everything himself, gave his famous advice: Divide the people into groups and then appoint aides to take care of their everyday needs. In essence, Moses was taught how to conserve his strength for the major decisions his subordinates could not make. Because the plan worked, Moses became one of the giant figures of world history.

Like Moses, classroom teachers face a multitude of responsibilities, problems, challenges, frustrations, and even failures. When dyslexia enters the picture, a teacher must accept help. Regardless of his or her enthusiasm and personal resolve, no teacher can possibly meet all the demands posed by the different learning styles in the classroom. Help must be found and accepted. It is not a sign of strength for harassed teachers to reject assistance in meeting the needs of disabled learners. In fact, it is difficult to defend a situation that pits a lone adult against the many needs of a roomful of students.

Using Older Students. One of the strengths of one-room rural schools was the interaction between older students and primary pupils. My own experiences as a student in a one-room country school have served as a lifelong model for behavior management. My teacher, Mrs. Kiethley, could have worked herself into an early grave had she attempted to teach all her students in all eight grades in that one large room. However, she demonstrated the wisdom of delegating responsibility. It was a special honor to be an upper classman in her school. When his or her behavior proved acceptable, an upper-grade student would frequently be called upon to "listen to little Johnny recite." This was a cue for the older student to take one of the little ones to the cloakroom, out to the shed, or in good weather down to the creek. There the upper-grade student would drill the younger student until the child was ready to recite for the teacher. It was old-fashioned but extremely effective in establishing accurate perceptual awareness of phonics, arithmetic, spelling patterns, history facts, or whatever needed to be mastered.

There was a double purpose in Mrs. Kiethley's classroom management, of course. She did not call upon only the better students to tutor. Quite often an adolescent boy, struggling with elementary reading or spelling skills, would be assigned the task of teaching the alphabet to a child in first or second grade. Or a 15-year-old might be called upon to teach multiplication facts to a 9-year-old. This pairing of tutor and learner was intended to reinforce the older student's skills as well as to accelerate the younger student's achievement. In other words, Mrs. Kiethley was practicing an age-old principle: *We learn much better the things we are required to teach to others.*

Many schools are remembering these old techniques in today's struggle to solve the dilemma of dyslexia in the mainstream classroom. By using older students as tutors, many teachers are finding a way to provide one-to-one attention for disabled learners. There is tremendous motivation for a sixth-grade boy to be asked to visit a primary classroom three times a week to teach a child the alphabet. Upper-grade teachers are witnessing changed attitudes in older students who now feel needed and involved, many of them for the first time in their school experience. It is impossible to say who benefits more, the tutor or the child receiving this individual attention. Both students tend to grow in academic skills.

Teachers have generally backed away from this sort of student-to-student teaching relationship on the grounds that only experienced teachers are qualified to give instruction. Although this may be true when teaching concepts, it is not always true that teachers are the best guides for skill practice. In fact, older dyslexics often are more effective tutors and monitors than professional adults. One dyslexic can express abstract ideas in a way that is quickly understood by another dyslexic child. Adults frequently find themselves unable to communicate so simply or so well.

An important two-way exchange occurs when an older student monitors skill practice with a primary student. First, an essential ego boost is gained by the older child who has struggled so hard and achieved so little. Being selected as a student aide usually does a great deal to awaken self-confidence and interest in learning. Second, the younger child is usually delighted and somewhat awed to have a "big kid" alone as his or her very own tutor. This is particularly effective when the older student is good at sports or has won some sort of public recognition.

The point is that harried teachers have a ready-made tutorial staff waiting to be recruited. Care must be taken, of course, not to use immature students who are not ready to handle a tutoring situation. If a personal clash develops, if there is lack of sufficient discipline, or if some other factor makes effective tutoring and learning impossible, then the relationship should be terminated immediately. Usually, however, enough capable older students can be enlisted to give every dyslexic child in the class 20 or 30 minutes of individual help two or three times each week. As Moses was relieved to discover, his new aides took much of the backbreaking labor off his shoulders. Then he was able to devote himself to the larger problems affecting the entire group.

Enlisting Adult Volunteers. National attention increasingly is being focused upon service to mankind, as opposed to satisfying one's own desires exclusively. Consequently, thousands of adults of all ages are donating a few hours each month to worthy causes. In every community there are interested high school students, housewives, working men with time to spare, and retired professional people who often feel unneeded by society. Schools near college campuses have still another prime source of energetic young talent, including future teachers. There is seldom any need for a classroom teacher to be overworked for lack of help. Assistance with teaching is more readily available now than at any previous time in our history. Teachers and administrators who have taken the initiative to enlist volunteer tutors have not been disappointed, as a rule. There is always some risk involved when outsiders are invited in. However, professional teachers usually do not find this to be a serious problem.

The main difficulties in enlisting volunteers are finding adequate space for one-to-one tutoring and having time to give the aides sufficient guidance about specific details of their work with children. Once these volunteers have settled into a regular tutoring experience, they need surprisingly little direct attention from the classroom teacher. They are monitoring basic skill drills, not teaching new concepts.

Parents of dyslexic children are among the most helpful volunteer aides. It is almost never wise for parents to work with their own children. It is a rare parent who can remain calm as his or her own flesh and blood struggles with symbol mastery. Emotions are too near the surface between dyslexic children and their nearest of kin. When this is taken into consideration, tutoring assignments can be made rather simply, so long as there is a relaxed relationship between adult and child.

Tutoring sessions need not take place at the school. In fact, it is often best for the child to leave school on released time, working at a nearby church, at the tutor's home, in a library, or some other place away from curious onlookers. Regulations governing student absence from school must be strictly observed, and this responsibility must be understood by the volunteer aides. Once these basic problems of time and place are solved, however, the tutoring sessions usually continue with no disruption of the classroom learning atmosphere. Responsible volunteers simply appear at scheduled times and the children leave quietly. Later they return without attracting attention. When a smoothly functioning volunteer system is at work, classroom teachers find many occasions to feel thankful and relieved. At last their struggling students are receiving individual attention. And at last they can devote their efforts to concerns that usually go unattended when the teacher tries to do everything alone.

Principles for Overcoming Auditory Dyslexia

Massive attention has been directed to the teaching of auditory skills, those skills that enable a person to identify specific elements of speech. It is theorized that once the learner can identify the component sounds of oral language, there should be little difficulty connecting written letters with the spoken sounds. In other words, if a student "hears" speech sounds accurately, he or she should have no trouble making letter/sound connections. Thus students are expected to learn to write the language they speak and hear. The reverse process is turning printed symbols into the oral language we speak.

On the surface this process of matching oral and written codes seems simple enough. After all, if students will only listen and pay attention, they can grasp the encoding and decoding processes which will lead into higher level reading ability. Armed with this assumption, authors, publishers, and classroom teachers have created mountains of materials and techniques for teaching "auditory acuity," "auditory discrimination," "phonetic analysis," or just plain "phonics." To the frustration of the profession, however, a sizable minority of students do not master these skills, regardless of the hours spent on phonics drill.

Most students who do not develop auditory discrimination are dyslexic. Earlier in this chapter auditory dyslexia was compared to tone deafness in music, meaning that the student does not "hear" differences between similar sounds in speech. This condition ranges from the inability to distinguish only two or three basic sounds to the inability to distinguish whole words. Some students confuse only a few short vowel sounds. Others recognize no vowel distinctions at all. The problem is not poor hearing. Instead, it is the inability to interpret what is heard.

Although traditional phonics instruction teaches most students to sound out words efficiently, phonics drill as it is usually presented is largely wasted on auditory dyslexics. If the tone-deaf dyslexic is to become a proficient reader and speller, different techniques must be used. Simply giving the tone-deaf student a stringent diet of phonics does not solve the problem.

A major factor in auditory confusion is the way phonics is presented in most reading programs. Only a few commercial reading programs begin reading instruction with carefully sequenced spelling patterns that follow the rules until the learner is confident enough to handle variations from the rules. Beginner students are usually faced with a conglomeration of whole words in which the letter/sound relationships are variable and inconsistent. It is not unusual for a beginner reader to see several spellings of certain vowel or consonant sounds in the same story.

For example, an auditory dyslexic would be frustrated by the following reading experience:

> "Run, Sue!" called Mother. "Here are four cookies for you."
> "Good-bye, Bootsy," Sue said to her doll. "I will eat a cookie for you."

In spite of weeks of drill on individual sound units, the dyslexic student is unable to cope with different spellings of the same sounds: run/Mother, Sue/to/you/Bootsy, for/four, I/Good-bye. The dyslexic learner is equally confused by different sounds for the same letters: run–Sue, Here–her, cookies–Bootsy, you–four.

It is virtually meaningless to a dyslexic student to be told, "Listen for the long vowel sound in *Sue.* Do you hear *u* say its name?" Usually the dyslexic does not hear the vowel at all. When the mysteries of decoding are presented in random order, the student with faulty auditory perception is lost from the start.

In seeking to remediate auditory dyslexia, parents and teachers must keep certain principles in mind.

Principle 1: Make Immediate Tangible Applications of Abstract Rules

Rules about phonics are almost always taught in the abstract, even when parents and teachers think they are providing simple, concrete illustrations for students. Adults are dealing in abstractions when they show the word *road* while emphasizing the "long sound of *o.*" When shown the word *road* and told, "Listen to *o* say its name," the student is confronted by three abstractions simultaneously: (1) the intellective act of attending to what the teacher says (tuning out distractions); (2) the printed word that represents the concept; and (3) the concept of "sound of *o* saying its name." Because they cannot filter out a single point from all the stimuli bombarding them, dyslexics cannot cope with even this simple cluster of listening/speaking/seeing relationships. The result is lack of comprehension of what the teacher means. What appears to an adult to be a very simple learning exercise is to dyslexic students a confusing jumble, a "roar," from which they glean no meaning. Consequently, the student fails to please the teacher, and another experience in failure has occurred.

It is difficult for parents and teachers to believe that older learners, even high school students or adults, may still need to work with concrete objects in order to nail down such foundation concepts as, "Listen to *o* say its long name." Even tone-deaf adults must experience beginning level activities, such as handling movable cutout letters, if they are to comprehend separate sounds in words. If auditory dyslexics are to master the foundation concepts of letter/sound relationships, they must experience immediate, tangible reinforcement. Teachers must realize that traditional reading instruction has not worked with auditory dyslexics precisely because there is not enough concrete reinforcement of abstractions. Regardless of the student's age, it is usually necessary to provide concrete handling experiences between sounds and letters.

Principle 2: Provide Multisensory Experiences

Most parents and teachers recall a concept from introductory psychology: *The more senses that are involved in a learning experience, the more fully the experience is learned.* This oversimplification of learning is a key to successful remediation of auditory dyslexia. If a student sees it, hears it, says it, feels it, moves it—even smells it or tastes it—he or she can begin to comprehend it. In other words, the more sensory channels that are utilized while learning, the more comprehension will be attained by the student.

There is some risk in overanalyzing (sounding out) words, particularly when dealing with isolated sounds and symbols. Some students misperceive, resulting in grossly exaggerated sounding out of words that makes reading impossible. For example, some students involved in phonetic reading programs that deal heavily with blending have the mistaken idea that each letter of the alphabet is a "word." *A* is "aye" or "a-aaaa," *B* is "bee" or "buh," *C* is "see" or "kuh," and so forth. It is perfectly natural, therefore, for such a student to perceive the word *cat* as three words, not three letters. Thus the student would drawl: "cuh-aaaaaa-tuh." Because this is like nothing heard in daily language usage, he or she completely misses the word *cat.*

Auditory dyslexics usually must begin with cutout letters, matching them, arranging them in sequence, and spelling out simple words the adult provides as models. Gradually, by using movable letters that students can feel, they begin to connect names and sounds to the letters they touch, feel, and manipulate. Many teachers have clinched such learning by adding taste and smell with cookies shaped like alphabet letters. The point is that whatever sensory stimuli are necessary to imprint the concepts within the learner's memory should be used.

For example, the only way auditory dyslexics can master phonics is to *see* the patterns rather than try to hear them. One of the most successful programs for helping tone-deaf students memorize phonics patterns is Glass Analysis. This program was developed by Gerald and Esther Glass and is published by Easier to Learn, Incorporated, P.O. Box 329, Garden City, New York 11530. Dyslexic students need to follow a five-step routine as they work through the Glass Analysis program, which requires approximately 2 years of steady practice: 1. See the word on the card. 2. Say the word aloud. 3. Spell the word aloud from memory. 4. Immediately type or write the word from memory. 5. Look at the card again to see if the student wrote it correctly. Over a period of time the Glass Analysis material covers all of the word family groups the student must know to read, spell, and write successfully. This kind of practice is excellent for the typewriter or word processor. The Glass Analysis cards can be used to build phrases and sentences as writing skills increase.

It has been pointed out earlier in this chapter that auditory dyslexics must see phonetic patterns in order to understand them. They cannot understand phonics just by hearing words or phonemes. Parents and teachers must follow a drill procedure that teaches the dyslexic how to combine several sensory pathways at the same time. The student must see/say/hear/touch all together. This is easily done by following a simple five-step procedure in drilling with visual phonics. For example, the adult makes a set of flash cards showing several words of the same family: *cat, bat, hat, rat.* Then the student does the following steps with each card:

1. *See the word.* Look at it. Touch it. Trace the letters with a finger.
2. *Say the word.* Say it from sight-memory, or sound it out if the student can. If he or she cannot say the word, then the adult pronounces it and the student repeats.
3. *Spell the word orally.* The student carefully says each letter in correct sequence while touching each letter to guide the eyes in refocusing correctly. If the student says any letters out of sequence, or if he or she calls a letter by a different name, the adult helps the student work out the correct spelling sequence. The student practices this oral spelling until he or she is sure that the word has been memorized.
4. *Type the word or write it from memory.* Without looking at the card, the student tries to encode it on the keyboard or with a pencil. He or she should whisper it as this writing is done.
5. *Check for accuracy.* After the word is typed or written, the student compares with the flash card. If any mistakes have been made, the procedure is repeated until the word can be encoded correctly.

This five-step visual phonics procedure moves slowly, and students can become bored doing this kind of multisensory practice. But this is the most effective technique for helping auditory dyslexics overcome their tone-deaf block in spelling. Over a period of time, this kind of multisensory drill with word family patterns will implant basic phonetic patterns within the dyslexic student's memory better than any other technique.

Principle 3: Provide for Kinesthetic Reactions

Many teachers control their classes by the dictum, "I want silence and plenty of it!" This mode of instruction is supported by administrators who judge the quality of teaching by the degree of silence in the classrooms. Unfortunately, a habitually quiet classroom is actually a poor learning environment for auditory dyslexics. Certainly the noise level must be controlled, but when body movement and vocal response are sharply curtailed, dyslexics are immobilized as essential learning channels are cut off.

During the 30 years I have worked with the dyslexic population, I have seen three basic behavior patterns found in every classroom (Jordan, 1977, 1988b). According to this system, three different styles of learning can be identified. *Number One* is the silent learner, characterized by a mostly passive, quiet, private manner that would delight old-fashioned librarians. Number One learners gain knowledge mostly through vision. They learn very well the silent way. During study time they want to be left alone. Number One's are seldom dyslexic, although occasionally we see disabled learners who fit this quiet, passive learning style.

Alongside the quiet students are the noisy *Number Two*'s. These students must combine three learning channels simultaneously to learn new information. They must see it, say it, and hear it all at once. If the noisy Number Two students are denied speech and hearing during study time, they do not completely internalize what is read. Number Two's can be forced into submission by overbearing adults, but they will always want to whisper or think each word while reading, which is an active substitution for saying it aloud. Noisy Number Two students usually drive the quiet Number One's up the wall unless the teacher takes steps to separate them during study time.

The remaining students are called *Number Three* learners. They are body learners who cannot cope with learning unless body motion and muscle reactions are involved. Number Three learners must see it, say it, hear it, and manipulate or touch it before mental images come together. When forced to sit still and be quiet, Number Three's cannot learn. These students usually become discipline problems in traditional classrooms and are usually regarded as hyperactive.

Auditory dyslexics are especially crippled when talking, moving, and touching are denied in learning situations. A remedial routine developed a generation ago by Lydia A. Duggins has been successful in awakening perceptual awareness of phonetic values in Number Three dyslexic children. The entire body is involved as the child bends, stoops, whirls, jumps, skips, or crawls, making the body act out the letter/sound relationships the child does not perceive through passive hearing alone. Dr. Duggins developed a five-step routine for teaching short vowel sounds. Donna, our auditory dyslexic example, stands *at* her chair for short *a*. She crawls *under* her chair for short *u*. She stands *on* the chair for short *o*. She sits on the *edge* for short *e*. And she sits fully *in* the chair for short *i*. As many clinicians have discovered, this kind of kinesthetic involvement is somewhat noisy, but it often works. When Donna's body moves in response to abstractions, she begins to understand what the phonics teacher is talking about. If auditory dyslexics are forbidden to use their overall body as a learning channel, being forced to sit passively and "think," the child cannot interact with the teacher's instructions. Rather than being a hallmark of good teaching, quietness is synonymous with illiteracy in the case of most dyslexics. Effective teaching means letting the dyslexic student be Number Two or Number Three. If this bothers Number One's, the groups should be separated when studying.

Principle 4: Build a Stock of Memory Cues

Even when they master the fundamental letter/sound connections for reading, auditory dyslexics usually do not become fluent spellers. This is because of their inability to retain clear visual images of word patterns. Because dyslexics do not "see" word forms when working from memory alone, they have no reliable memory cue system for accurate recall of word patterns. In other words, when there is no visual model to see, the auditory dyslexic is helpless to reconstruct accurate words on paper.

Adult dyslexics who have achieved academic success have done so by devising their own systems for recalling specific spelling patterns. Few dyslexics ever tell about their private memory tricks for fear of being thought silly. It does sound strange to listen to a dyslexic whisper while working out spelling patterns: "Let's see . . . 'mother' is *t-h-e* with *mo* in front and *r* on the end . . . 'warm' is *a-r-m* with *w* in front. . . ." Because they cannot "see" sound patterns in printed symbol form, auditory dyslexics remember bits and pieces of spelling patterns, tacking on letters to flesh out the skeletal structures as they are recalled.

When parents and teachers are aware of this perceptual need, they can help dyslexic students a great deal. After assigning the week's spelling words, the teacher can help learners like Donna devise whatever meaningful memory cues they can handle. It is completely irrelevant whether a dyslexic student's memory tricks make sense to the adult. The important thing is whether these tricks help the student. If the learner *needs* memory tricks, then anything else is irrelevant and should be disregarded in the interest of achieving literacy.

Principle 5: Emphasize Consistent Spelling Patterns

An old-fashioned technique that is regaining acceptance is to drill with word families. This introduces children to stable, similar patterns that stay with the rules. Many teachers have used this technique under the guise of "consonant substitution." The device is to present a root spelling, such as the *at* family. Then students practice building familiar words by placing different consonants in front of *-at: cat, bat, hat, rat.*

Many teachers shy away from nonsense words (e.g., *lat, wat,* or *dat*). However, many dyslexic students are delighted with nonsense word forms. In fact, most youngsters spend a great deal of their private fantasy time devising word games. In a form of solitaire, they mimic words they hear, creating nonsense vocabularies just for the fun of it. Successful teachers know that making nonsense words is a highly motivating activity for many reluctant readers and spellers.

Even adolescents respond well to this activity, so long as the teacher turns a deaf ear to the double entendre items that inevitably occur. If things become too earthy with street-wise adolescents, the teacher should stop the double talk at once. This is done by informing the culprits: "I know *exactly* what that means, and I don't want to hear it again." Before calling a student's bluff, however, the teacher must be sure the student is consciously trying to be cute. Some naive youngsters (as well as parents and teachers) have no idea that their words or phrases carry double meaning.

The important point is not to confront dyslexic students with variable spellings that violate the rule they are trying to comprehend. For example, if Donna is coming to grips with the fact that when *o* comes by itself inside a short word, it has the sound of *o* in *hot,* then she should not suddenly be exposed to the word *cold.* It is totally irrelevant at this point that "*o* before *ld* has its long name." This kind of generalization has no meaning to most dyslexics. Their mastery of letter/sound connections is built upon visual cues, not upon abstractions. In fact, even intelligent adult dyslexics seldom become skilled with phonics rules. Teachers of dyslexics must realize that these unique students seldom respond to abstractions. Instead, learning procedures must be structured around a system of memory tricks and visual cues. If the classroom can provide for this unorthodox learning style, much can be done to help auditory dyslexics compensate for their perceptual deficiencies.

Principle 6: Provide Visual Cues

A firmly entrenched attitude among parents and teachers is that tests must be taken strictly from memory, if we are to determine just what the student has learned. Consequently, all visual cues to answers are removed, forcing students to retrieve information or organize responses from memory alone. This rather curious custom is unfair. Taking tests from memory arbitrarily labels talented test takers as "good students," while those who perform awkwardly on tests are called "poor students." Those youngsters who are gifted with quick, accurate memory (retrieval) are the star performers, regardless of whether they can make practical application of their knowledge. In fact, the term "test wise" is often heard among educators, denoting the students who know how to pass tests, even when they do not understand the content of the questions. Also in current use is the cynical student phrase "multiple guess," referring to the so-called objective tests that force students to select one of several arbitrary choices.

Forcing dyslexic students to work from memory alone when their memory (retrieval) is erratic is certainly questionable educational practice. When such a student can function well if given visual models for points of reference, then it is imperative that teachers provide this kind of reinforcement.

For example, it is not cheating on a spelling test when Paul glances at the cursive writing chart to remind himself of how to write a certain letter. This is survival. Neither is it showing favoritism for the teacher to display model spelling patterns while the class is doing written test items. If navigators need trustworthy directional instruments to point the way to specific destinations, dyslexics must have visual cues. The purpose of education is to produce independently literate individuals who know how to read the signs and do what they say. Dyslexics are placed in hopeless situations when teachers hide all the visual indicators, forcing the students to work from memory. The same teachers would be horrified to see a track coach confiscate the crutches of a physically disabled boy, then force him to hobble after his able-bodied peers just to "test" his track skills.

Visual cues can be in the form of pictures, graphs, charts, colors, or textures—whatever is appropriate in the classroom situation. Regardless of the visible code, auditory dyslexics prove remarkably knowledgeable when allowed to work where they can see visual reminders. Without such reinforcement, they become understandably restless, uncooperative, and eventually hostile toward school.

Principle 7: Allow Oral Answers to Test Questions

Parents and teachers who read this book can recall personal experiences of frustration in taking an examination. Teachers and college professors are aware of the near panic felt by many adult students, including teachers taking graduate courses, when they are forced to work strictly from memory in answering comprehensive test items. Physicians who practice near universities know when qualifying exams are scheduled for doctoral candidates. Medical clinics are besieged by graduate students seeking relief from hypertension, ulcers, and near collapse under the strain of taking tests without benefit of visual cues. It is unfortunate that adults who experience such trauma seem to have so little understanding of the feelings and needs of children.

Dyslexics show the same behaviors as worried adults at test time. When required to write what they should have learned, working entirely from memory, they face a difficult choice: They can either endure the pain and embarrassment of flunking another test, or they can avoid the test if possible. This intense frustration causes much of the ugly classroom behavior seen in dyslexics who decide to fight the system. This sort of confrontation is not necessary.

When alternative ways to respond to tests are provided, dyslexics usually exhibit satisfactory knowledge. Through listening and even reading, struggling students gain a great deal of accurate information. Classroom teachers who understand the dyslexic dilemma have discovered that these students can be held responsible for specific information if allowances are made for their handicaps in reporting or writing. Oral tests have proved the answer for many struggling students. When they are tested orally without being penalized for their dyslexic handicaps on paper, these students experience success, which, of course, is what education is all about.

4

Overcoming Dysgraphia

Handwriting is a sensitive personal matter. Under certain conditions graphologists may introduce handwriting analysis as court evidence because a person's penmanship is a unique signature of the writer's personality. Partly because of this personal nature, penmanship practice has been one of the least popular school activities, especially for boys. In recent years educators have removed pressure from children to make their handwriting perfect. Students no longer have to fill pages with the push-pulls and smoke screens that are remembered well by older persons. More teachers are accepting uniqueness in children's writing, so long as the writing is legible.

It might be helpful to point out a technical difference between *dysgraphia* (inability to write legibly with a pencil or pen) and *dysorthographia* (inability to spell correctly from memory). Many poor spellers develop good enough penmanship to win praise for their handwriting, yet they never master basic rules of spelling. This poor spelling pattern has been described in previous chapters. On the other hand, it is not uncommon to find good spellers who cannot write legibly. The struggle to write clearly (dysgraphia) often masks adequate spelling ability which emerges when the poor writer uses a word processor. The struggle to spell accurately with a pencil or pen (dysorthographia) is not always related to poor penmanship.

Ironically, old-fashioned penmanship drills may have corrected a form of dyslexia which is a serious educational problem in modern classrooms. Since the introduction of manuscript printing in primary grades, many intelligent youngsters have not learned to write acceptably. Fifty years ago penmanship drills saturated children with perceptual awareness of letter formation. Today thousands of students are failures at handwriting.

The inability to cope with handwriting is called *dysgraphia*. This term refers to difficulty in producing legible handwriting. Dysgraphia involves faulty control of the muscle systems needed to write letters and words accurately. The dysgraphic student usually has a clear mental image of what the left brain intends to encode, but the student keeps "forgetting" how to write specific symbols. Certain letters are made with backwards or upside-down motions. Handwriting is generally so awkward and unsatisfactory that dysgraphic students try to avoid situations that require them to practice penmanship.

Many dysgraphic persons learn to read. However, dysgraphia is usually associated with both visual and auditory dyslexia. Teachers and parents seldom see one form of dyslexia that is not complicated to some degree by other signs of impairment. When seriously dysgraphic students are permitted to use alternate means of writing such as typewriters, word processors, or dictation machines, handwriting disability can be largely ignored as an educational problem. So long as educators insist that all students master manuscript and cursive styles, dysgraphia will continue to be a frustrating educational handicap.

Dysgraphia Syndrome

It is important that teachers distinguish between careless handwriting habits and perceptual impairment. Boys often reject the restrictions of attractive writing style. Since teachers tend to judge student competence by the neatness of written work, dysgraphic students are at a serious disadvantage. There are definite characteristics that differentiate dysgraphia from carelessness. The problem is not difficult to diagnose, in view of the wide variety of handwriting samples available from each student's written work every day. The following sections describe specific characteristics associated with dysgraphia. Appendix 3 contains a checklist of symptoms to look for.

Difficulty Learning Alphabet Forms

The primary characteristic of dysgraphia is the student's difficulty remembering how to write certain letters. The classroom teacher might not identify this flaw unless he or she watches the student write. Cursive writing style is intended to flow from left to right. Dysgraphia involves the tendency to work backwards, from right to left. So long as primary pupils print isolated letters in manuscript style, this backward tendency may not be a major problem because the letters are not connected in a series. Dysgraphia becomes a crippling factor as children are expected to develop skill in left-to-right cursive writing style, usually taught in third grade.

Few adults are aware of the staggering perceptual burden modern education has placed upon beginner pupils when it comes to writing the symbols of our language. Adults who have good literacy and handwriting skills think that children have to master only 26 alphabet letters. Unfortunately, this is not true. Since the early 1930s American educators have taught manuscript print in kindergarten and first grade. Yet the alphabet is seldom taught in sequence (A through Z). Instead of learning only 26 letters, primary students are expected to master two sets of alphabet symbols, including capital and lowercase, for a total of 104 alphabet letters. Since many manuscript capital letters are distinctly different from lowercase letters, the beginner student must learn 52 letters in manuscript style, not 26. Later, when the transition is made to cursive style, 52 new letters must be learned, bringing the total to 104.

Manuscript print is usually continued throughout second grade. All of this time young readers are exposed to a wide variety of type styles in their reading materials, on television, in magazines, and so forth. The Library of Congress lists more than 100 typefaces commonly found in reading materials in America. Near the end of second grade or by the middle of third grade, children are told that manuscript style will no longer be satisfactory. Now they must forget all that they have learned about print writing. Now they must master a new style of letter writing. The 52 isolated, unconnected manuscript letters mastered through years of drill are now gradually discarded while a new handwriting style, called cursive, is introduced. As with manuscript print, cursive style utilizes not just the 26 basic alphabet letters but 52 new forms, although several capital and lowercase letters are similar. By the beginning of the fourth grade the primary pupil is expected to have learned to write 104 alphabet forms from memory. This includes unlearning 2 years' work spent mastering the concepts of manuscript letter formation.

Along with learning to cope with 52 manuscript symbols, primary students are simultaneously confronted by more than 30 printer's cues commonly used in basal readers, library books, textbooks, and other sources of reading in elementary classrooms. Youngsters are expected to distinguish several marks of punctuation, color cues, boldface type, italics, indentation, chapter and story headings, unusual page format, and other symbols included in the repertoire of beginning reading skills. These symbol systems take on meaning only when students have successfully mastered the relationships of the symbols to the students' speaking and listening language. Few adults would willingly attempt such a staggering burden of symbol mastery within a 3-year span. The wonder is not that many children fail; the wonder is that so many succeed. To start a child's quest for literacy with manuscript printing is a serious barrier for handicapped children who are more confused than edified by 104 alphabet symbols within a 3-year span.

Dysgraphia becomes a crippling factor as it brings the student into conflict with tradition, particularly the left-to-right pattern of reading and writing. Cursive letter forms involving closed, circular strokes are difficult for dysgraphic children. Equally difficult are letters requiring a change in direction of hand movement. Dysgraphic writers frequently have problems remembering where to stop a sweeping or circular movement, how to swing back, and how to connect the lines of movement within complicated letter formations. They have great difficulty remembering where and how to stop circular motions in order to swing accurately into the next letter when writing words. The difficulties are dramatically reduced when children are taught cursive style instead of isolated manuscript printing.

Teachers and parents must develop two skills of observation if they are to detect dysgraphia quickly. The teacher must actually observe the student at work. Dysgraphic writers often mask their difficulties so that the handicap may not be apparent on sample papers the teacher collects for evaluation. It is also essential for the adult to learn to re-create the student's writing style by tracing over the student's handwriting slowly, observing the flaws in directionality and discovering where the writing breaks down.

Figure 4.1 is a sample of writing by an intelligent girl in fourth grade. This was Glenda's attempt to write the alphabet from memory. This illustrates her confusion in transferring from manuscript to cursive style. She mixes the two styles in her writing. Dysgraphia is noted by her difficulty forming the loops on *d, b,* and *p.* She also confuses *d* and *b* because of her initial experiences with these letters in isolated, unconnected manuscript style. Capital *Z* causes Glenda considerable confusion, as indicated by her erasures and awkward overprinting. By tracing over her writing, the reader can feel the dyslexic confusion Glenda experiences.

Dysgraphia is easily seen as parents and teachers review children's written work. Figure 4.2 shows a spelling test by a fourth-grade student. Any example of writing can be used to look for dysgraphia. The reader should slowly trace over the writing, saying the words over

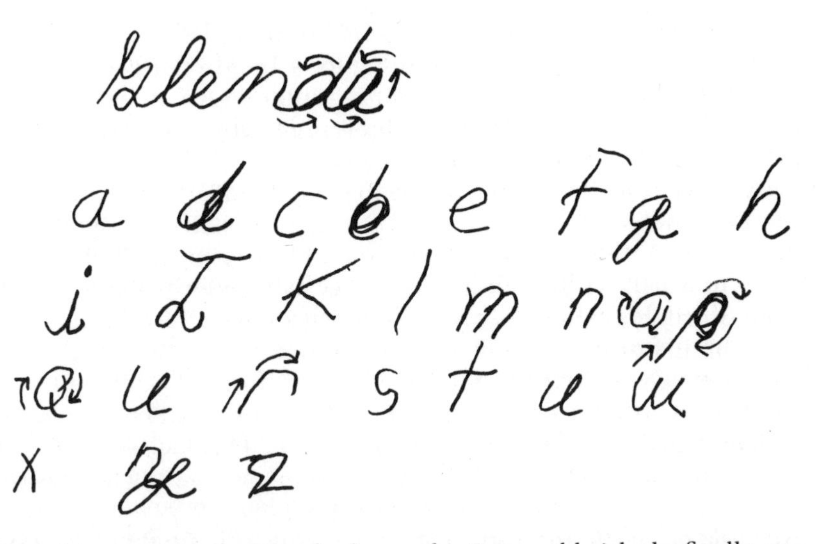

Figure 4.1. A writing sample of a dysgraphic 9-year-old girl who finally mastered good cursive writing skills by learning the D'Nealian technique of continuous stroke writing. The small arrows show direction of stroke.

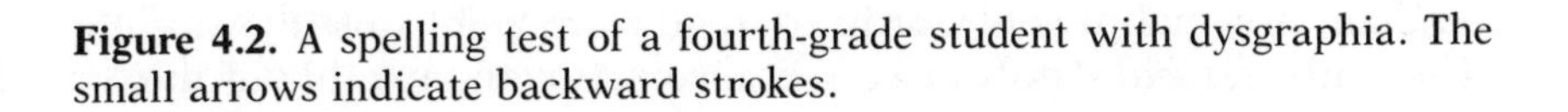

Figure 4.2. A spelling test of a fourth-grade student with dysgraphia. The small arrows indicate backward strokes.

and over while tracing, just as the student mumbled the words as he or she wrote. The small arrows in Figure 4.1 and Figure 4.2 indicate the backwards strokes these dysgraphic students use in writing. This chronic reversed hand stroke is the reason why such students are extremely slow, insecure writers.

A careful observer will note the many broken letters in Figure 4.2. This boy's writing is actually a series of pieces strung together. In words like *pig* that begin with *p*, the child starts at the bottom and marks upwards, ending in a backwards loop to form the top of the letter. Since this causes the writer to finish the pencil stroke inside the letter, he is forced to break writing continuity by starting the next letter somewhere near the bottom loop on *p*. Initial *f* is often patched together because the dysgraphic writer does not recall how and when to change the direction of the pencil motion. This lack of continuity causes the dysgraphic writer to circle again and again when writing *d, b, a, o,* and *e,* as illustrated in the words *barn, brown, party, duck, bear, doll, ate, goes,* and *play*. The reader can easily imagine the panic this child experiences during pressured writing activities in school.

A more serious form of dysgraphia is illustrated in Figure 4.3 in the writing of a highly intelligent boy in third grade. This student's work is handicapped by a combination of visual dyslexia and dysgraphia, as revealed by the reversed letters and word elements. These dyslexic tendencies were almost entirely corrected during a 14-week cycle of intensive training which supplemented his regular classroom activities. The key to success was his mastery of D'Nealian cursive writing, an excellent writing program published by Scott, Foresman and Company (Thurber, 1984). The child practiced an hour each day until he had mastered the cursive lowercase alphabet in D'Nealian style. As alphabetical order and sequence became automatic, the dysgraphic problems shown began to disappear. By the end of third grade this boy was meeting grade-level expectations in writing and spelling from dictation.

Mirror Writing

An interesting form of dysgraphia is commonly called "mirror writing." True mirror writing can actually be read when held up to a mirror. A complete mirror image is rarely seen by parents or teachers, but varying degrees of this tendency are commonly found in dysgraphic work. As a rule, only certain words or portions of words will be written backwards. The counterpart of mirror writing is mirror reading, in which whole words are read from right to left ("was" for *saw,* "tub" for *but,* "no" for *on*). Figure 4.4 is an example of mirror

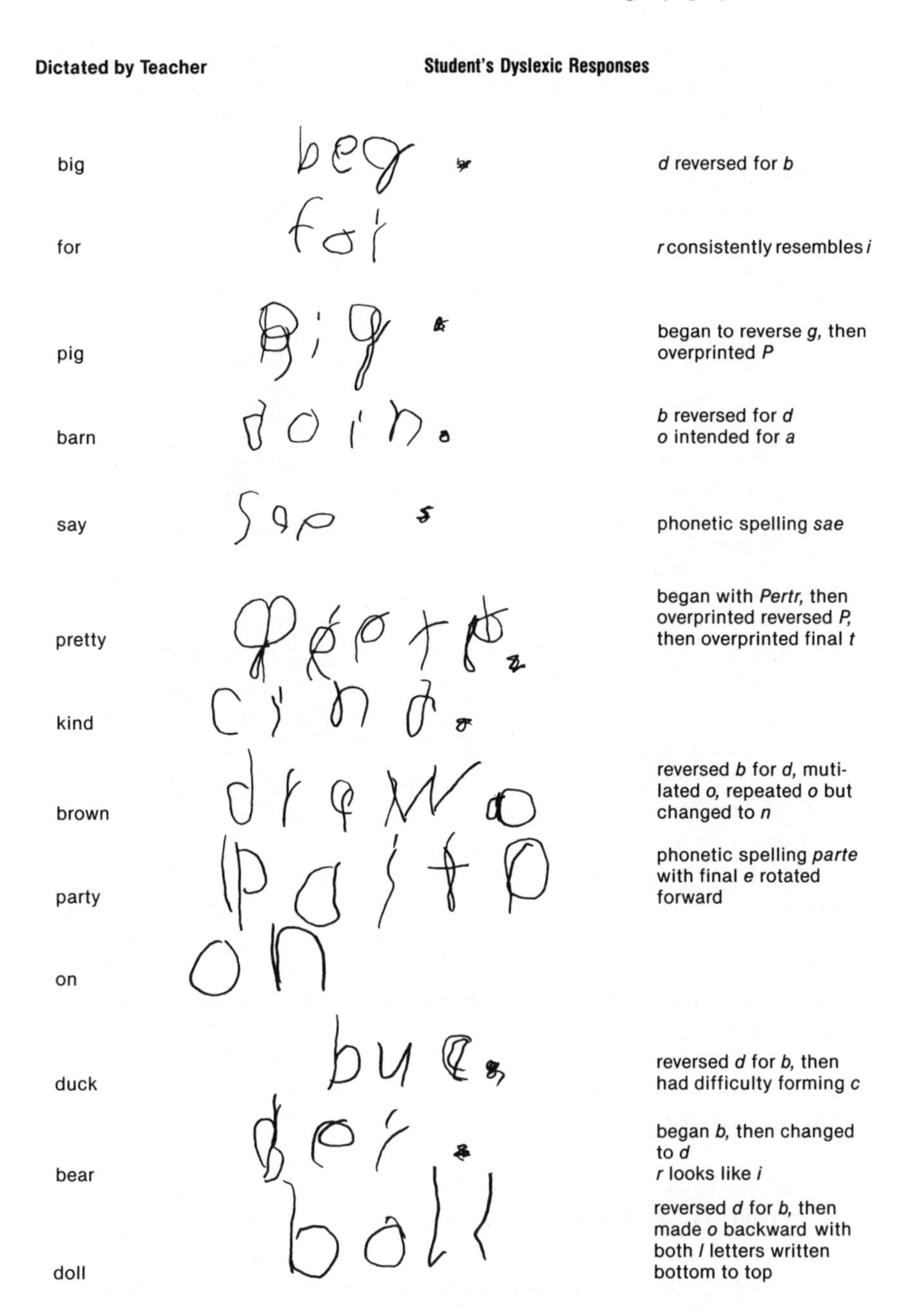

Figure 4.3. A writing sample of a third-grade boy with combination visual dyslexia and dysgraphia.

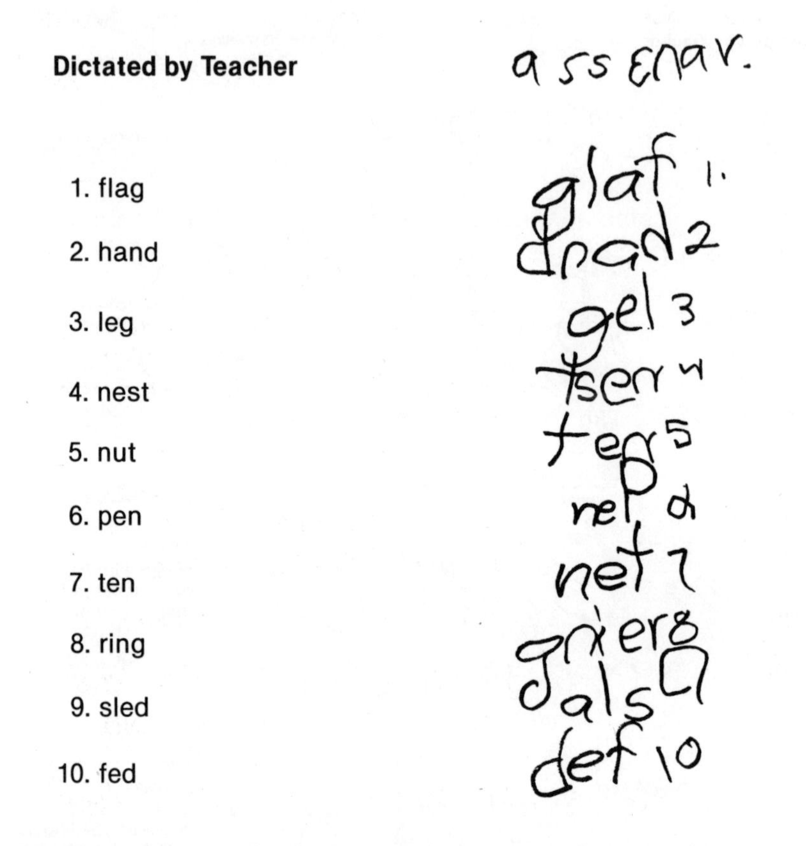

Figure 4.4. An example of mirror writing produced by a student in second grade.

writing done by Vanessa, a bright child in second grade. She did not exhibit mirror tendencies in reading. Because she had partially adjusted to left-to-right sequence, she was able to overcome her tendency to mirror write rather quickly when the teacher understood the nature of the handicap.

Scrambled Sentence Structure

A significant clue to a dysgraphic student's language potential is sentence structure, or syntax, which is largely camouflaged by poor handwriting. Two examples of frustrated creativity are presented in Figure 4.5 and Figure 4.6. The passages have been translated to illustrate the language maturity of each child. In each case an interested teacher

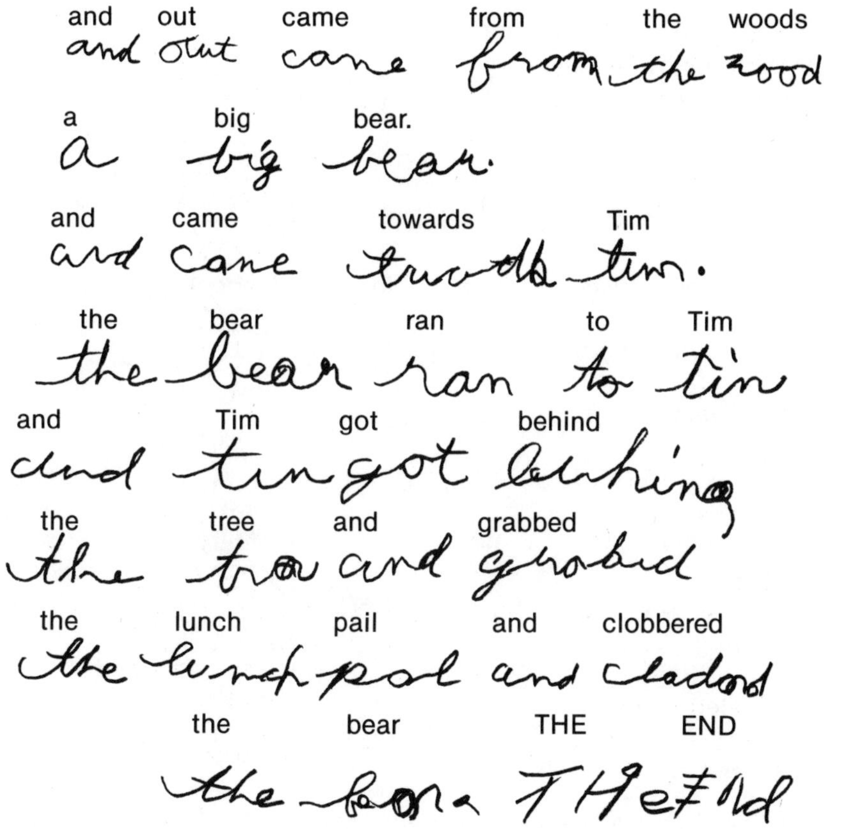

and out came from the woods

a big bear.

and came towards Tim

the bear ran to Tim

and Tim got behind

the tree and grabbed

the lunch pail and clobbered

the bear THE END

Figure 4.5. A dysgraphic student's response to an unfinished story. The sample shows language maturity that is masked by poor handwriting.

took time to decipher the messy, crudely done handwriting which at first glance seemed not worth wading through. When the perceptual impairment had been recognized, these children were no longer regarded as lazy and careless. They made rapid progress by mastering the D'Nealian writing style.

The first example (Figure 4.5) is Donna's response to an unfinished story in her reading class. After reading a brief story about children picking blueberries and being startled by "a loud, astonishing noise" from the woods, she was asked to imagine what happened next and then write an ending in her own words.

Andrew's Christmas story (Figure 4.6) represents a near tragedy in misdiagnosis according to surface evaluation of standardized scores. The Wechsler Intelligence Scale for Children–Revised

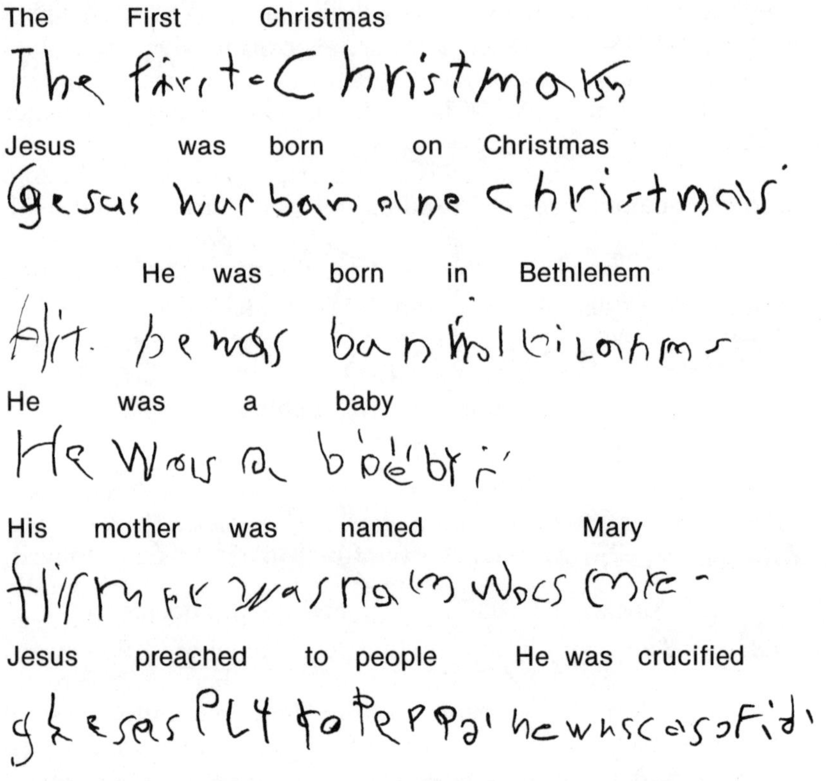

The First Christmas

Jesus was born on Christmas

He was born in Bethlehem

He was a baby

His mother was named Mary

Jesus preached to people He was crucified

Figure 4.6. A sample of a dysgraphic student's poor handwriting. Based on test scores that showed no impairment in coordination, this student was originally misdiagnosed as severely emotionally disturbed.

(WISC-R) yielded Verbal IQ 103; Performance IQ 110; Full Scale IQ 107. Andrew achieved Motor Age Equivalent 8.0 on the Bender Gestalt Test, 6 months above his chronological age. The Human Figure Drawing Completion Test yielded a score of 101 at the 53rd percentile level. However, Andrew's handwriting was virtually illegible in daily classroom work. The psychometrist concluded that a severe emotional disturbance must exist. After all, it was reasoned, the motor indicators on the clinical tests "ruled out any sort of impairment in coordination."

This rigid reliance upon test scores was challenged by Andrew's classroom teacher, who had noted a sophisticated language structure in the child's work. A reading diagnostician identified the problem as dysgraphia, which does not always show up on clinical tests for motor development. Older students helped the classroom teacher guide Andrew through daily training in D'Nealian handwriting skills. Within 6 weeks his dysgraphic symptoms had begun to disappear. This incident illustrates the danger of professionals looking more at scores than at actual classroom performance of children.

The major flaw in Andrew's manuscript print is the broken letter pattern. Lowercase *a, h,* and *m* are usually fragmented, with the strokes scattered apart. This gives his writing the appearance of "bird scratches." Several letters are rotated toward the left, adding to the disoriented appearance of his work. These faults were quickly remedied as he mastered the D'Nealian writing style.

Poor Directionality

A crippling aspect of dyslexia is the inability to see how parts of a whole pattern relate to everything else in the pattern. For example, students are expected to read horizontally from left to right. In writing, the right-handed student is supposed to progress horizontally from left to right with the page tilted slightly toward the left. If a page is divided into columns, the student is expected to progress downward until the eyes or hand reach the bottom line, then move directly upward and to the right for the next column. Since our literacy system is based upon the left-to-right, top-to-bottom orientation, anyone who perceives reading or writing differently is "wrong." Students with poor sense of directionality do not automatically interpret book pages or work pages in this standard way. They continually lose their place and need guidance to follow left-to-right, top-to-bottom format.

Left-handed writers frequently develop a legible writing style, although they often appear to write upside down or backwards. This unorthodox compensation of "lefties" has frustrated many parents and teachers who feel that correct pen-to-shoulder alignment is a sacred ingredient for sound scholarship. But in a largely right-handed world, left-handed students have been forced to develop their own unique writing styles, protests from traditionalists notwithstanding.

A subtle but common problem associated with dysgraphia is confusion with horizontal and vertical directionality. Occasionally, totally inverted perception is seen by clinicians. Such individuals read exactly upside down, perceiving symbols at 180 degrees rotation from "normal." Because these students are usually capable readers, their upside-down orientation is often not discovered until they have to write. Teachers frequently see certain students turning the reading page halfway around. This indicates that the child perceives at 90 degrees rotation. For these readers the print becomes legible only when the rows of words are vertical. This rotated orientation usually disappears as children are indoctrinated to "correct orientation." The tendency seems to bother adults more than it does the child.

Directional confusion does create a problem in handwriting, however. This form of dysgraphia is frequently camouflaged by extremely poor letter formation or by the messy appearance of the student's papers (see Figure 4.6). As the dysgraphic student attempts to write, particularly with no visual model to copy, directional confusion creates jerky production with much erasing and writing over. The writing usually cuts through the line or wobbles up and down about the line. When moving from the bottom of one column to the top of the next, the writer sometimes switches to mirror image, writing on the left-hand side of the midline instead of on the right.

Difficulty Copying Simple Shapes

An earmark of dysgraphia is the inability to copy simple geometric shapes without distortion. This is often referred to as conservation of form. Teachers assume that students can hold mental images of what they see while those images are translated through fine muscle coordination onto paper. Dysgraphia is the inability to do this complex perceptual task. Parents and teachers can use any activity involving copying circles, squares, diamonds, triangles, or rectangles to see how well a child can do this simple work. It is important to allow for immaturity in younger children in primary grades. Dysgraphia is indicated only when other symptoms are also present in the child's handwriting. The Jordan Written Screening Test (Jordan, 1977, 1988b) identifies this dysgraphic tendency.

Figure 4.7 demonstrates how a simple copying activity reveals dysgraphic tendencies. This work was done by a boy in sixth grade, age 12 years, 9 months, with mental ability within the average range.

A frequently observed flaw in copying shapes is the tendency to draw "ears" on the corners of simple figures. Parents and teachers can see this tendency on arithmetic pages and art activities which ask students to sketch or copy shapes and figures. Figure 4.8 shows examples of "ears" that indicate left-brain inability to handle right-brain images, not low intelligence.

Telescoping

When dysgraphic students are laboring to write longer words, they commonly leave out portions of the letters or syllables without being

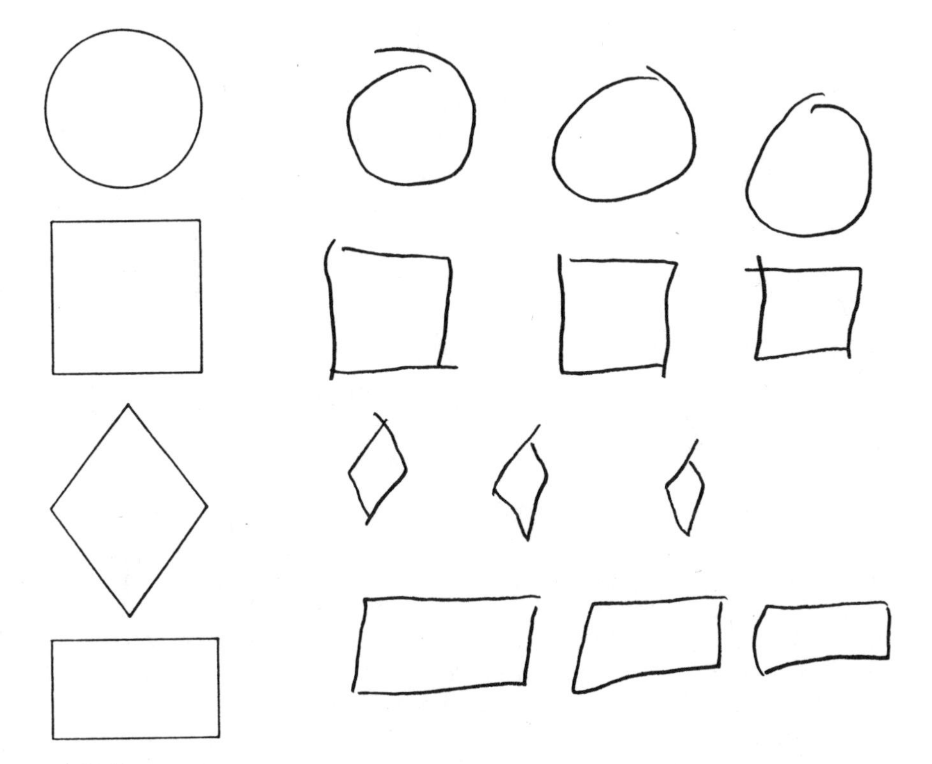

Figure 4.7. A copying activity revealing dysgraphia in a sixth-grade boy.

aware of this error. The effort of putting word units onto paper is a labored process for dysgraphics. After writing for a brief time, they start to lose track of how much of a word has been encoded. This habit is called telescoping and is illustrated in the spelling errors in Chapter 3 under "Sound Units Omitted." Students who tend to telescope are usually handicapped by auditory dyslexia as well as dysgraphia.

Perseveration

The opposite of telescoping is perseveration. This problem involves the inability to turn loose of a pattern once the student has begun to produce a certain sequence. Perseveration is sometimes heard in oral reading or conversation when the speaker repeats vocal patterns unnecessarily. Occasionally perseveration occurs during rhyming drills, as when a student responds to *cat* by saying: "vat, dat, lat, nat, wat." This usually is not an effort to be amusing. True perseveration

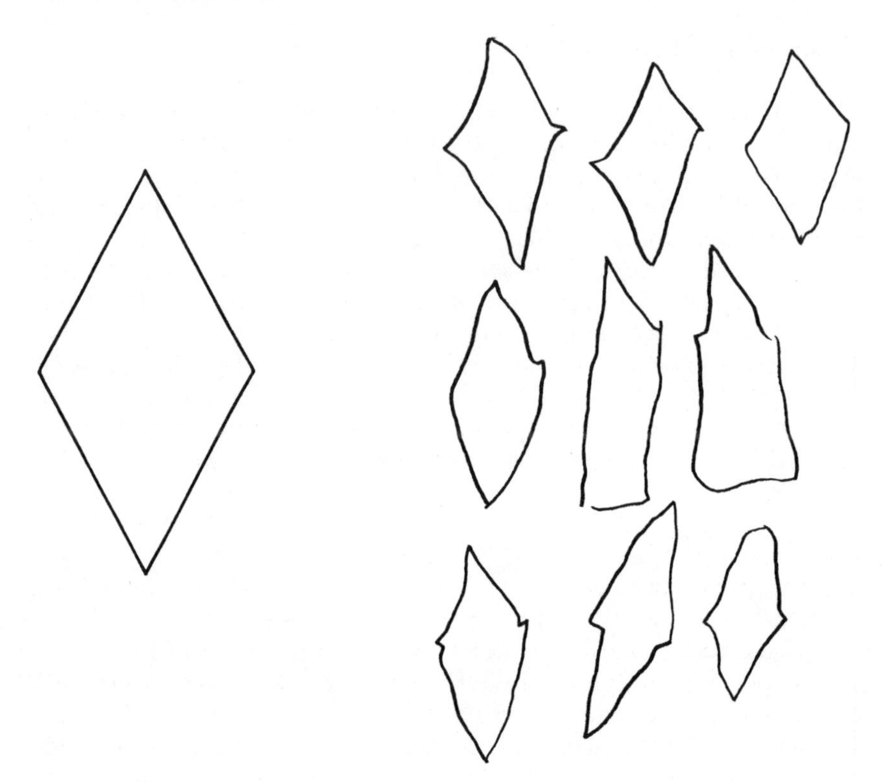

Figure 4.8. Copying activity showing "ears" on corners, revealing dysgraphia.

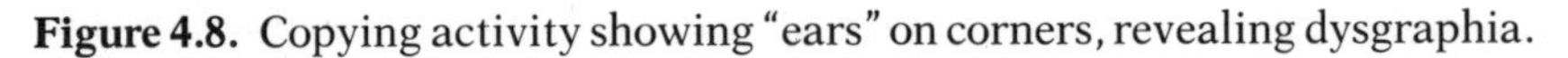

is an involuntary reaction. The person is momentarily unable to stop the repeating reflex.

Dysgraphic writers are often unable to halt the reproduction of certain letter or syllable patterns without completely stopping their writing, then starting again. Perseveration also results when the writer habitually lifts the pencil from the paper midway through writing a word. This break in continuity leaves writers unable to recall where they stopped in the word pattern.

Activities for Overcoming Dysgraphia

The following sections describe activities that can be used in the classroom to overcome dysgraphia, including activities dealing with directionality, handwriting, poor eyesight, dictation, checking for errors, and increasing work output.

Establishing Directionality

The primary disability underlying dysgraphia is the inability to deal with directionality. This means that when the writer attempts to write symbols on the page, he or she does not have a clear, automatic habit of proceeding from left to right or from top to bottom. Instead, the writer tends to mark circular strokes clockwise, which is backwards from what educators call correct. The dysgraphic writer also tends to start at the bottom of the letter or numeral and mark upward. Again this is backwards to standard orientation.

There is nothing wrong with backwards orientation as such. If left alone to adapt to reading, writing, spelling, and arithmetic in their own way, most dysgraphic students would devise ways to cope with literacy requirements in our culture. The major obstacles around which they cannot move are stereotyped expectations which parents and teachers hold regarding handwriting. When these artificial penmanship restrictions are laid aside, the dysgraphic student becomes as able as most others to do the work of an educated person.

The school's hostility toward those who deviate from the norm inflicts permanent damage in dyslexics. By the time dysgraphic children reach middle elementary levels, their interest in developing writing skills has either been extinguished, or they have become too defensive to respond to usual classroom procedures. The fight to preserve private territory (individuality) has absorbed all of the student's time and energy. There is little inclination in older dysgraphics to develop the niceties of "correct" writing. Handwriting has been perceived too long as the enemy responsible for their rejection by adults and classmates. Dysgraphic youngsters are among the most seriously damaged casualties of our educational system. Overcoming their disabilities is a long-range undertaking, but it can be accomplished in most cases.

If parents or teachers wonder whether this description of the dysgraphic's plight is overly dramatic, they should listen as these children verbalize their feelings to counselors and tutors. Visual and auditory dyslexics appear to enjoy school, compared to most dysgraphic students. The difference seems to lie in attitudes of parents and teachers. Most youngsters can at least trace adequately or draw acceptable pictures, thus gaining a degree of respectability. But the dysgraphic child who cannot coordinate the writing process is without even these means of gaining acceptance. Not only does Donna have difficulty reading and spelling, she compounds her struggle by being messy with her work. Correcting dysgraphia calls for a great deal of patience on the part of the adult. Not only must the instructor teach writing skills, the teacher must also convince children like Donna that it is safe to try.

Mastering Handwriting Skills

Regardless of the student's age or grade placement, there is an essential starting place to correct faulty concepts of directionality in writing. The student must begin with cursive writing. This proposition flies in the face of educators who for half a century have preached that manuscript printing must come first. The reader should keep in mind that this book concerns exceptional children, not those who fit the mold of the majority. Since most children do prosper by learning manuscript printing first, there is no intention of upsetting their educational routine. But if dysgraphia is to be corrected, cursive writing style is essential, regardless of whether the learner is 5 or 50 years of age.

There now is available to parents and teachers one of the most effective handwriting programs we have seen in several decades. A creative elementary school teacher and principal, Donald Thurber (1984), realized early in his classroom experience that dyslexic/dysgraphic children could not do their best with the traditional "ball and stick" manuscript writing form, then change to cursive writing later on. Thurber developed a new handwriting system based upon single-stroke pencil movements instead of the isolated ball and stick pencil movements that are so difficult for many children. This new approach to writing is now published by Scott, Foresman and Company as the D'Nealian writing program (Thurber, 1984). (The title D'Nealian is an acronym devised from Thurber's own name: Donald Neal Thurber.) Many dysgraphic children, adolescents, and adults are now writing legibly with great pride, thanks to the creative work of Thurber. The D'Nealian system of writing gives the student a simple, dependable way to write in cursive style with only a few instances where the pencil has to be lifted and replaced to make certain letters. Single-stroke writing is solving penmanship problems for a new generation of students who cannot master handwriting skills in the traditional "ball and stick" way.

Coping with Poor Eyesight

Dysgraphic students often have major problems with vision control. Certain characteristics of letter formation, irregular spacing, ragged left margins, telescoping, loss of place, and poor placement of writing on the page often signal problems with eyesight. Teachers often see dramatic disappearance of dysgraphic symptoms when faulty vision is corrected. Students who cannot control binocular visual movements or who cannot maintain clear focus in sustained work are handicapped in copying, doing workbook assignments, and handling writing activities. The teacher must make sure that students can see well enough to do written work before assuming that learning disability (dysgraphia) is the cause for poor penmanship.

Practicing Dictation

The goal of most teachers is for the dysgraphic child to learn to write clearly and with reasonable accuracy when taking dictation or writing from memory. This ability cannot be developed in one school term by a single teacher, except in some cases with adults. Weekly spelling words provide an ideal channel for emphasizing dictation writing skills. When working with dysgraphic students, the teacher must let them know ahead of time what they will be expected to write. This means that elementary teachers should begin giving one or two brief sentences which will be dictated at a specified time. It is important that this dictation effort *not* be graded. This is a training procedure, the purpose being to teach the dysgraphic child to cope with more complex dictation in later years. During the year the teacher should expand the quantity of dictated material until the dysgraphic student is able to cope with five or six full sentences at one sitting. This kind of structured drill will increase the student's confidence in writing from memory without having models to copy.

Checking for Mistakes

An essential survival skill for dysgraphic students is knowing how to edit their own written work for errors. This is an especially sensitive area of corrective teaching because dyslexics often react strongly to criticism. The teacher must provide ample opportunities to let students check their own work against whatever model is being used. It is particularly helpful for students to check any work for which a grade will be given. Spelling tests, arithmetic assignments, social studies exercises, or science quizzes are suitable for this purpose. If dysgraphic children are taught how to use answer keys or other scoring devices, they will be able to protect personal territory and pride by being the first to see their failures. Once the errors have been checked, the student does not mind so much if the teacher or other students see the work. The damage occurs when apprehensive writers turn in work that they suspect is not perfect. Suspense builds up to painful peaks before the paper is returned. If indeed it has not been good work, the student's ego is torn once again by the red ink all over the paper. Checking one's own work first is a face-saving device that is very important to insecure learners.

There is no greater risk of cheating among dyslexics than among honor students. In fact, cheating is almost always a direct measure of the pressure a student is under to be accepted by the system. If parents or teachers discover dishonesty as students do self-checking, the adults should reexamine their values regarding the importance of grades. The presence of cheating is usually a reliable cue that too much emphasis has been placed upon achieving good grades. Insecure students resort to cheating to find acceptance within a learning situation. If the pressure is coming from the child's home, the teacher's options are limited. Aside from counseling such a child, there may be little the teacher can do to relieve anxieties about grades. If the pressure is from within the school, the grade standards must be adjusted for the sake of the child. There is great value in having dysgraphic students monitor their own work for mistakes, both to preserve private territory against outside criticism and to see one's own progress, or lack of it. It is a regrettable educational loss when self-criticism must be denied because students cannot be honest with themselves without feeling rejected by the system.

Increasing the Quantity of Finished Work

Regardless of the parents' or teachers' good intentions, no student can be fully protected. Sooner or later dysgraphic writers must cope with arbitrary demands for finished work when no consideration will be given to their problems. Eventually students must either cope with doing written assignments or drop out of the system.

Raising Production Quotas. It is not difficult for parents and teachers to map out production schedules for dysgraphic students. This is best done on thermometer charts that resemble the large outdoor signs used to show how fund-raising campaigns are progressing. Movable colored strips are raised by degrees to indicate new writing quotas that the dysgraphic student is expected to reach. By using color codes along with other symbols, each writer's production goals are constantly shown. Each week the teacher reevaluates each student's work. If dysgraphic youngsters are making sufficient growth, their quotas for the coming week are increased by a small amount. If a particular writer has not yet conquered a specific dysgraphic problem, the quota remains unchanged. Occasionally the expectation must drop for someone who has become discouraged. The point is to cause learners to stretch in small increments to make sure that steady growth is maintained.

The key to growth lies with the parent and teacher who must sense when quotas are reasonable, or when too much is expected. If the student accepts the new goals in stride, all is well; he or she is ready to meet the higher output schedule. If frustration and signs of insecurity emerge, the new goals are too high. The student's reaction to the thermometer chart is usually a trustworthy indicator of how ready he or she is for higher productivity.

There need not be a great deal of bookkeeping involved in maintaining production charts. If the student is working in three major areas—reading, writing, and arithmetic—then the production chart should have three thermometer columns, each equipped with a color strip that moves up or down to indicate changes in the teacher's expectations. Each column is labeled at the top by whatever subject the writer is working in. Up the side of the chart are numerals, with lines running across the face of the chart.

For example, if Wayne is expected to finish three written papers this week, the colored strip under Writing would be raised to line number 3. If he is also expected to finish five papers for Math, that strip is positioned at line number 5. If for Reading he is to turn in four written assignments, that thermometer strip would rest on line number 4. Thus a clear visual monitor has been provided for Wayne as well as the teacher. On Wednesday the teacher can safely ask how he is coming on his weekly work schedule. By comparing the number of finished papers in his folder with the color code on the chart, both Wayne and his teacher have an instant check of how much more work must be done before Friday afternoon.

Dysgraphic writers like Wayne can be held accountable for meeting their quotas, because this kind of visual cue system is fair. The student knows on Monday exactly what the teacher expects for that week. The teacher is relieved of trying to remember these details, because Wayne's assignments are reflected on the chart. The contract with Wayne to honor his territory by not nagging him to do his work is able to stand. By reminding him each day to check his own progress, the teacher is avoiding the danger of trespassing on his inner space, which occurs so commonly in the classroom. On the other hand, Wayne has no excuse for failing to meet his production schedule. This is a fair way to teach dysgraphics how to accept increasing amounts of responsibility. If they "goof off" during work time with their responsibility fully in view, they must suffer the consequences. As part of the working agreement, students already know what the consequences will be. The teacher has already informed them of the penalty for failing to carry out the contract.

This sort of visual contract is as effective in kindergarten as it is in high school. In fact, for many years industry has used similar systems of production reminders for adult assembly workers. Employees who receive incentive pay according to their output are far more productive than those who receive only a base wage. Parents and teachers who work on a contract basis, giving worthwhile rewards for acceptable work as well as significant penalties for work failure, have been amazed at the differences they see in student attitudes.

It is hard work to nag students into doing their tasks. The clever parent or teacher utilizes incentive programs that do the nagging. In a way, the production chart is harder for the student to ignore than the nagging voice of the adult. There is something about the silent, persistent presence of a quota chart that spurs most learners on to fulfillment of their obligation. This sort of self-discipline is critical for the dyslexic. Lifelong lessons in timing and self-programming are instilled when dysgraphic children are held accountable by a production chart. When Friday afternoon comes, there is no way they can escape the truth. If the week has been wasted, then the student must face judgment. If the week has been spent productively, then the student receives the reward.

The quota chart also allows the parent or teacher to present alternatives. It is especially important for dysgraphic students to be allowed a choice of written assignments from which they can make a selection to submit for evaluation. If Wayne has done several more papers than the chart requires, he should be allowed to hand in the papers he considers best for the week. Thus both student and teacher are allowed to save face. When given this opportunity to decide their own fate, dysgraphic writers cannot blame the teacher for low marks on their work. In turn, the teacher is free to make whatever candid suggestions are necessary. When the full decision has been the teacher's, both adult and student are placed on the defensive.

Probably the most important learning derived from a quota system is self-discipline. Of all students in our schools, dyslexics usually are the least self-controlled. Their entire perception of life is a scrambled blur of events, pressures, obligations, and information, much of which appears disorganized and incoherent.

Without a highly structured system that keeps their lives ordered, dyslexics seldom achieve a sense of well-being. Dyslexic adults who have succeeded in spite of their handicaps have learned how to order their circumstances.

It would be tragic if dyslexics were taught only how to read, write, spell, and do math. Their primary social need is for self-control, which of course includes literacy. Production schedules are essential for students who cannot comprehend chronological time lapse. If these young people are to manage family budgets, job responsibilities, and leisure activities well, they must be taught the ingredients of self-control over a period of several years. This is one of the major contributions parents and teachers make in correcting dyslexia.

Keyboard Writing. During the past few years new technology has opened the door to good writing for dyslexic/dysgraphic students who are handicapped with penmanship and paper and pencil tasks. Keyboard writing is rapidly becoming accepted by parents and teachers as an answer to their problems with these struggling writers. A remarkably effective touch typing system is now available, designed specifically for dyslexic children. The *Type-Write Program* (Johnson & Stetson, 1984) was initially developed by Imogene Johnson at Central State University in Edmond, Oklahoma, because of her own son's dyslexic needs. Later Johnson was joined by Elton Stetson at the University of Nevada in producing the *Type-Write Program.* This simple program first teaches the student to match fingers with keys on an electric typewriter. Then the student works through a systematic review of the basic spelling patterns, sight words, phrases, and sentence structures found in daily school materials. Every student who finishes the *Type-Write Program* shows improvement in spelling, ability to write good sentences and paragraphs, and reading comprehension. Word analysis skills (sounding out words) also improve because of greater attention to left-to-right sequence and to all of the important details within words.

Once the students have mastered the keyboard through the *Type-Write Program,* they are ready to begin writing with a word processor. Many microcomputer systems now offer self-correcting spelling programs that catch spelling mistakes as the student taps out the message on the computer/word processor. In the near future several word processor systems will also offer programs that will catch mistakes in grammar and punctuation. Tomorrow's writing will be vastly easier for dyslexic students, now that these keyboard writing systems are available. Within a few years dyslexic students will have small, portable word processor units that can be carried to class in briefcase-size carriers. By the time today's elementary students are in high school, a new world of keyboard writing technology will be available to let them produce the good written work they are capable of if penmanship is not a consideration. New word processor technology will do for dysgraphic writers what hand calculators have already done for math students. Soon there will be no reason why parents and teachers cannot provide this excellent technology for dyslexic/dysgraphic students who heretofore have been seriously handicapped in producing written work.

Principles for Overcoming Dysgraphia

In spite of recent prophecies that a new day is coming when handwriting will be obsolete, classroom teachers are still very much concerned with a student's ability to communicate in written form. It may be true that today's primary students will function in an adult world where machines will do the encoding. Meanwhile, it is essential that students develop enough handwriting skills to cope with the world of today. The ability to put one's thoughts into legible written form is still a live issue in the classroom.

As described earlier in this chapter, the dysgraphic writer like Andrew usually has an idea of what he or she wants to write. The student may even have a model from which to copy. The disability is that he or she cannot manage to put an acceptable written code on paper. Handwriting is flawed by broken letters. The student cannot recall whether to move the pencil to the right or left. Instead of beginning at the top of a letter to make a down stroke, this writer starts at the bottom and marks upward. Circular motions go clockwise, which is backwards. In putting thoughts into writing, the dysgraphic student tends to run letters together, telescoping until entire syllables are obscured or omitted altogether. At times this writer perseverates, repeating writing motions or letter shapes until the written work is nonsense. Occasionally a dysgraphic student will be unable to make legible letters at all, filling the page with "bird scratches" that make sense only to the writer. Regardless of how hard students like Andrew try, they cannot satisfy adults because of their awkwardness doing handwriting.

Correcting dysgraphia in the classroom is possible if certain principles of instruction are observed. The classroom teacher must keep in mind that dysgraphics are not just being messy or disrespectful. Unless these students have become bitter and hostile through repeated failure, they will tend to do their best each time they write an assignment. The teacher holds the key to the child's attitudes and self-concept. If the student does his or her best, but it is never good enough for the teacher, then serious damage will occur in exactly the same way that damaged feelings occur when adults are forced to work for impatient, critical supervisors who are never pleased. If the classroom teacher can practice patience and long-range optimism, success can be realized over a period of time.

Principle 1: The Student Is Doing His or Her Best

I learned a painful lesson about dysgraphia the second year I taught school. My sixth-grade students were asked to write stories built around "trigger words" written on the chalkboard. Wayne seemed especially interested in the project because the trigger words suggested a science fiction theme, his favorite fiction form. I graded the stories with my usual thoroughness, marking every spelling, grammar, punctuation, and penmanship error with a blood-red pencil. Wayne's story content was unusually good, but the mechanics were awful. At that time I had no knowledge of dysgraphia. My attitude was that every student could do good work if he or she tried hard enough. I handed back the papers at the end of the school day, then dismissed the class. As Wayne passed me, I saw tears in his eyes. "I liked your story," I said. "Then why did you bleed to death all over it?" he sobbed, running from the room.

As a teacher I had failed to understand a vital fact: *Wayne had done his best.* The messy, smudged paper I had rejected was the best he could do at that time. In "bleeding" all over his mistakes, I had failed to perceive that he had done his best for me, and I had rejected him. His best was not good enough for my standards.

Like most proficient grown-ups, parents and teachers tend to think of children as miniature adults. This frame of reference blinds us to many vital elements in educational growth. Because we assume that what we see is what really exists, our children are judged by the surface characteristics of neatness, punctuality, quietness, dignity, poise, and how well their work fits the mold. The stereotypes by which we judge student achievement can be cruel, if we mistakenly assume that imperfect papers are evidence that the child has not tried. Such rigid expectations may have some validity for children without disabilities. However, sensitive students like Wayne are hurt day after day, year after year, because their inability to fit the mold brings false judgment upon them. The truth is they usually try harder than their peers who always make good grades.

How does a classroom teacher or parent determine whether children are doing their best? The only feasible way to make such a judgment is to note indicators of improvement. For example, if

Wayne has always disregarded (failed to perceive) small details in copying from the board or from a book, his work would have poor punctuation, failure to indent for paragraphs, disregard of capital letters, and chunks left out. The adult will know Wayne is doing his best when he begins to perceive the minor details that affect comprehension. In other words, improvement must be judged by the small corrections students begin to make on their own, after these deficiences have been pointed out by the teacher. If over a period of time there are fewer and fewer mistakes, this is proof a student is doing his or her best.

An essential factor in correcting dyslexia is mercy. Although mercy, patience, understanding, and forgiveness are not directly related to phonics or word analysis, these attitudes are of critical importance in the classroom treatment of dyslexia. The merciful teacher is one who begins to look for bits and pieces of improvement, instead of continuing to "bleed to death" over the multitude of errors. It is difficult for some adults to believe, but when Wayne begins to observe capital and lowercase letters, this represents a tremendous stride in achievement for him. What might be an inch forward for the teacher may represent a hundred feet of progress for the dysgraphic child. It is cruel and harmful to judge progress always by large increments. If children must leap all the way from C to B to demonstrate that they are doing their best, there is no hope for the dyslexic in the classroom. When teachers can accept the small tokens of progress as being giant steps for the dyslexic, then mercy will begin to heal bitter attitudes, allowing additional progress to be made.

The first step toward correcting dysgraphia is not more handwriting practice. The first step is for the adult to believe that even the messiest, grubbiest papers may represent the best the student can do under the circumstances. In other words, the adult must forgive the student's deficiences. Far too many adults are biased against dysgraphic writers solely because their written work is messy. Once it is recognized that the student is actually doing his or her best, then it is time to work for improvement.

The secret is to scan the dysgraphic student's work for molecules of improvement: certain letters no longer reversed; punctuation marks now being used; capital letters where they are supposed to be. Many teachers have reversed their marking systems, using the student's favorite color to mark only the points of progress. A paper with no marks would signify no improvement. From this point of view, Wayne would cherish the days when the teacher marks up his work, heralding the fact that at last an adult sees improvement.

Principle 2: Handwriting Is Intensely Personal

It would be profitable if every parent and classroom teacher could relive his or her most sensitive experience in which personal writing was criticized. Adults, especially teachers enrolled in graduate education courses, are extremely sensitive when their written efforts are being judged. Any professor who returns research papers, essay test responses, or written reports can testify to the acute pain experienced by adults who find critical notes on the margins of their work. It is not unusual for grown-ups to burst into tears over criticisms professors have made. The point is that none of us is immune to feeling sensitive about what we have written. Editors are especially aware of the problems new writers face in learning how to accept editorial suggestions. Of all the sources of dread that professionals feel, having one's writing criticized, misunderstood, or belittled is among the most acute.

This universal sensitivity toward one's written work is reflected in the way adults carefully guard personal diaries and intimate letters. Although school work is by no means as personal as one's private notes, there is a common feeling of caution when people are required to commit themselves to written form. Oral communication is not remembered verbatim, and the speaker's clever use of intonation and mannerisms can distract listeners from any personal revelations that might be uttered. But thoughts put into writing become permanent. In writing, an intimate part of the writer's self becomes vulnerable once it is encoded upon the page for all the world to see.

Sensitive adults are aware of how this timidity in writing affects classroom behavior. From the earliest grades through graduate school, insecure students slip up to the teacher to ask: "Do you want to see what I wrote?" Teachers do great damage when they impatiently send these students back to their seats without glancing over the written material. Professors who do not take time to scan a nervous graduate student's first draft inflict similar pain. When students reach out this way, they are actually pleading: "Please don't be too critical. This is the best I can do. Is it good enough yet?"

As students achieve success, they need less reassurance from parents and teachers. Repeated success with writing, especially if one has language gifts, brings enormous satisfaction. Teachers always look forward to having students who write well with an interesting style. But this kind of success is seldom available for the dysgraphic child. Since dyslexics are by nature overly sensitive, they often compensate by appearing indifferent to praise. In reality, they are hungry for the acceptance experienced by more able learners. When forced to commit themselves to written form, dyslexics have no defenses left. Writing becomes a threatening experience. If the classroom is geared to the high levels of penmanship usually expected by parents and teachers, the weaknesses of disabled writers are fully exposed. Their choice is to muddle through, like Wayne, or to grow so defiant that they refuse to try. If they hand in their messy papers, the teacher "bleeds to death all over them." If they choose not to try, then they are publicly branded as lazy, careless, uncooperative, or even "dumb." No matter which way they turn, they lose, according to their point of view.

The dysgraphic problem has been intensified by the educational stereotype of correct penmanship. In reality there can be no such thing as the "correct" way to hold one's pencil, or slant the paper, or sit in one's chair while writing. Neither can an adult logically dictate the angle at which another's letters must slant, nor the balance he or she should obtain between ascenders and descenders or circles and loops. The penmanship standards demanded by educators have been arbitrary, based more upon bias than upon perceptual reality.

In recent years handwriting has come to be recognized as a unique signature of the writer's personality. Wayne slants his letters toward the left, not because he is "incorrect," but because of unique tendencies of his individuality. The size of the writer's script can have a definite correlation with his intelligence, just as the way he or she dots *i*s and crosses *t*s indicates specific character traits or dispositions of mood. It is terribly presumptive for a parent or teacher to declare that a child is "wrong," just because the child's script does not flow like the adult's. A great deal of ignorance has been involved in handwriting methodology, especially where dysgraphic children have been concerned. Fortunately, the term *correct* is being supplanted by the more realistic term *acceptable.* Having one's best efforts accepted does not imply that further progress is not needed. But being labeled *acceptable* allows room for growth, a step at a time.

If writing is indeed a highly personal thing, then parents and teachers should handle the subject accordingly. The rule of thumb should be a practical one: *So long as the student's writing is legible, and so long as it is the best he or she can do under the circumstances, I shall accept it without making him or her feel inferior. Gradually the student will learn to write more acceptably in order to avoid embarrassment as he or she matures.*

Principle 3: Respect the Student's Territory

A few years ago the world of anthropology was startled by a dramatist who became a popular science writer, Robert Ardrey. In two fascinating books, *African Genesis* and *The Territorial Imperative,* Ardrey elaborated upon the research of Dr. S.V.E. Leakey, who spent his life tracing mankind's origins in Africa. Ardrey drew hundreds of examples from the animal world to support his thesis that human beings, like lower animals, possess a strong territorial imperative that we will defend at all costs. Ardrey contended that this instinct to stake out one's territory, and then defend it against threatening intruders, explains human behavior. According to his idea, every aspect of human civilization—religion, education, politics, family, recreation, technology, war—is governed by the need for territory. From his observations Ardrey inferred that, to be a wholesome individual, every person must have a certain degree of privacy (territory) in which the person is safe from intrusion by outsiders. The theory holds that, when human beings are deprived of private territory, they become neurotic, ceasing to be emotionally well-balanced.

This idea has been explored by scientists like Konrad Lorenz, who raised various kinds of animals, observing and defining their territorial behavior. Studies like these have suggested some useful applications for education. There have been excellent learning results where territorial needs have been provided for in teaching situations. Regardless of one's opinions about the conclusions that writers like Ardrey draw, there is an immensely important lesson for teachers and parents in the concept of territoriality in the classroom and at home.

If adults are to help strugglers overcome learning problems, then close attention must be given to the interactions between frightened, insecure dyslexic students and confident, sometimes overbearing adults. Few teachers or parents realize that one adult alone with one child is rarely a one-to-one relationship. If the adult is overbearing and the student is insecure, the relationship is often overwhelming for the student. This explains why some struggling learners do not respond to private tutoring with some adults. When viewed through the perspective of territorial imperative, dyslexic behavior does indeed appear defensive because the disabled learner feels his or her territory (inner privacy) is threatened. This accounts for much of the disruptive behavior encountered by teachers of learning disabled students. Most adults do not hesitate to defend their rights (territories) against outside threats. Walkouts, strikes, professional holidays, and other forms of protest have become common among educators. If professional adults react in this fashion when their territories are violated, then certainly one would expect overly sensitive dyslexics to do the same.

The classroom incident with Wayne illustrates this principle. As his teacher, I had carefully "motivated" him to respond to the creative story assignment. I want to say that I coaxed him out of his shell. What actually happened was that he let me enter his private world of make-believe. I was proud of the expertise with which I manipulated the whole class into writing stories from the trigger words. After all, did they not decide to use my words instead of theirs? Until I saw Wayne's angry tears, it did not occur to me that I had made an unspoken contract with my students:

> "If you will write a story as I've suggested, I'll read it carefully. I know it's hard for you to spell and punctuate accurately, but don't worry about that. The main thing is for you to express yourself—be creative! You can trust me to appreciate the part of yourself you put down on paper. I won't betray your trust!"

Then I "bled to death all over it," as Wayne so well expressed the situation.

The fact that I was a young teacher was no excuse for my violation of this dyslexic boy's trust. As a sensitive adult, I certainly knew the pain and embarrassment of having my own writing (territory) violated by stern graduate professors. Not 6 months prior to that day with Wayne, I had driven home in tears of rage because a professor had belittled a paper I had written for his graduate course. The mistake I made with Wayne was not to respect his territory. I betrayed his trust by "bleeding" on his mistakes, and then I compounded the injury by saying, "I liked your story." He reacted as any healthy person should react by thrusting me out of his inner territory. It was several weeks before he let me back in. There are times when classroom teachers never regain a comfortable relationship with students whose territories they have failed to respect.

If parents or teachers are to gain entry into the inner space of dysgraphic children, they must establish ground rules that will govern the behavior of both parties. This is sometimes called a contract. Basically the teacher has a frank, private conversation with the dyslexic student, explaining the skills that need to be developed. The teacher presents a checklist of the trouble spots in the student's work, along with samples of work to illustrate these deficiencies. Then the teacher proposes alternatives, naming the kinds of activities available for correcting the problem, specifying the amount of individual attention he or she can give, explaining the grading system, and telling who the aides or tutors will be, if such help is available. At first not all students are mature enough or interested enough to receive all this information. The adult must use good judgment to determine when enough has been discussed at one conference. The point is to present a simple outline of the student's needs, explain what can be done about it, and specify the student's responsibilities in overcoming the problems.

There are many reasons why a student like Wayne might be reluctant to admit the teacher into his confidence (territory). In the first place, he probably will not trust the adult to keep the bargain. A wise teacher does not push to get in. There is nothing more devastating to struggling learners who have trouble expressing ideas than for an articulate, outgoing adult to bombard them with personal questions. The adult should not try to pry answers from the student. If no interaction is forthcoming, the adult should take the initiative by making direct statements on how, when, and where the corrective work will begin. As students gradually digest the teacher's offer to help, they will realize that the instructor is genuinely ready to accept them, weaknesses and all. At this point they will begin to open up in conversation. In fact, one of the dilemmas of tutoring dyslexics is how to persuade them to stop talking in order to accomplish drill work.

The gist of this principle is simple and direct. The parent or teacher must not overwhelm the student, entering private personal territory before the student is ready to accept the adult there. Until the learner gives cues that he or she is ready for a more personal relationship, the adult must confine outward interests to simple drill routines, explaining whatever the student seems interested in knowing. Above all, written work must not be condemned, even when it is illegible. The adult must devise tactful ways to require unacceptable work to be done again. This is best done by letting students evaluate their own work against a model. Above all, the teacher must not "bleed" all over written papers to the point where students feel discouraged.

When the parent or teacher genuinely respects territorial boundaries, and is careful not to betray the subtle trusts students begin to show, then great strides toward improvement are seen. Abrupt, impatient, and domineering adults see virtually no growth among the dyslexics in their charge. Such strong personalities usually do not realize the effect they have on sensitive students. Most domineering adults perceive themselves as excellent teachers because their rooms are quiet and their students busy. Such teachers should never be in charge of dyslexics. Territorial boundaries are so fragile in these children that a heavy-footed adult tramples down the fences many times each day without realizing the inward devastation such forceful behavior is causing. In other words, teachers should be chosen for corrective work because of their skills in sensing the territorial boundaries of sensitive students. Strong-willed adults should be placed with outgoing, competitive students who thrive upon competition for territorial dominance in the classroom.

5

Overcoming Failure and Developing Self-Confidence in Dyslexics

The most critical problem with which a dyslexic person must deal is stress. From the first experiences with language until the end of their lives, language disabled persons wrestle with the ever-present factor of stress. The left-brain dysfunctions described in chapters 1 through 4 are operative from early childhood as the youngster tries to comprehend oral language, remember things accurately, and interpret the hundreds of signals that must be understood if one is to be a functional member of society. As Chapter 3 described, dyslexic children continually mishear, misperceive, misinterpret, and misunderstand the complex world in which they live. Being dyslexic means experiencing the never-ending stress of trying to do one's best, but continually disappointing key people in one's life. The chronic social and academic stress experienced by dyslexics is similar to living with chronic pain. On better days the pain can be ignored, but it is still there whenever the body moves a certain way. On better days dyslexic persons can almost forget their language dysfunction, but it is always there, ready to trip them up without warning. This continual haunting background of language disability colors all of the dyslexic person's relationships a certain shade of gray. As the dyslexic child matures into adolescence and as the adolescent becomes an adult, this chronic pressure from stress takes its toll. Self-image, self-esteem, and self-confidence must grow in the rocky soil of never being free from the arid influence of stress.

To understand how stress influences dyslexic persons to such a great degree, we must review our scale of severity:

0	1 2 3	4 5 6 7	8 9 10
none	mild	moderate	severe

In earlier chapters we have seen how dyslexia ranges widely from being mild (merely an occasional nuisance) to severe (a serious disability). Stress follows this continuum closely. A person who occasionally reverses certain symbols, tangles the tongue in saying longer words, misunderstands several words that sound alike, and must consult a dictionary to make sure certain words are spelled correctly will feel stress from time to time. These episodes of stress come more through frustration with self than from outside pressure. This mild level of dyslexia triggers frequent flashes of irritation. Occasionally it brings a rebuke from a teacher, parent, or boss who complains about the dyslexic "blips" that cause errors. This kind of stress comes and goes. It is embarrassing and frustrating, but it is not chronic or severe. Persons who have only mild (occasional) dyslexic patterns can usually handle this degree of stress, although we sometimes see an overly sensitive person blow this kind of periodic stress out of proportion. With friendly counseling, most persons who are mildly dyslexic handle their stress with no ego damage resulting.

Stress becomes a problem when dyslexia is within the moderate range of severity. As we have seen in earlier chapters, persons who are Level 5, 6, or 7 on the severity scale make continual mistakes. Spelling is never fully accurate. Details in sequence are continually scrambled or cluttered. Listening comprehension is faulty and creates a lot of misunderstanding. Reading is usually slow and labored. It is hard for these dyslexics to take accurate notes rapidly enough to keep up with a flow of new information. They get body-in-space directions confused or reversed (east/west, north/south, left/right). They continually "forget" important things unless they keep lists and daily schedules in writing. They tend to be late for meetings and appointments. They are usually slow doing certain kinds of activities that require recall of specific information. They tend to lose their words as they speak. They forget the names of people and cannot always remember what to call familiar objects. They lose their words as they tell or describe. These persons are awkward, hesitant, slow, and prone to make careless mistakes, when they are compared with others their own age. Moderately dyslexic children, adolescents, and adults live under a constant weight of stress because they do not fit the expectations of their culture. They almost never find safe places or circumstances where they are completely accepted without some kind of judgment or criticism entering the relationship.

Dyslexics at the severe level live in a constant state of heavy stress. Few persons at Level 8 or 9 on the severity scale know what it is to be free from social, educational, economic, or family stress. The occasional Level 10 dyslexics often do not survive without serious mental health problems because their developmental years have been so saturated by stress that crushes their ego structures. Severely dyslexic persons grow up within a cloud of constant criticism. They are never free from being reminded "You messed up again!" or "Why don't you ever try to do it right?" or "Don't you ever listen to what I tell you?" If parents happen to be compassionate and supportive, teachers often are not. If a brother or sister seems to understand, grandparents or other relatives may not. If one boss is tolerant and forgiving, other bosses are not. If the severely dyslexic adolescent or adult exposes himself or herself to the risks of romance in dating, they run the extremely high risk of being rejected, once the special friend finds out. Dyslexics with severe handicaps in reading, spelling, speaking, and slow work pace face especially traumatic situations trying to find work. If they reveal their dyslexic condition, few employers will hire them. If they tell a military recruiting officer about being dyslexic, they usually will not be admitted into military service. If they say much at all about being dyslexic, they are told, "Well, we all have our problems," or "You just use your dyslexia as an excuse." These handicapped persons frequently meet adults who believe that dyslexia is linked to mental retardation, or that there is no such thing as dyslexia. Everywhere severely dyslexic adults turn, they face the stress of either dealing with the problem alone or being rejected and criticized because of it. From the earliest years when toddlers begin to interact with their larger world, dyslexics feel the stress of being different and not being correctly understood.

No human being can develop normally and wholesomely if he or she cannot find some freedom from stress. In those who are not dyslexic, stress takes a heavy toll in heart disease, digestive problems, anxiety, mental health breakdown, ruptures in personal relationships, and so forth. It is impossible for anyone to be a whole person if stress exists day after day, year after year. The irony of dyslexia is that the problem that triggers stress cannot be removed through counseling or therapy. This chronic life pattern is built in before birth, or occasionally it is caused later by injury to the brain (trauma-induced dyslexia). Because dyslexia is a brain-based dysfunction, it will always be there to some degree. Dyslexic persons must develop ways to cope with their chronic patterns so that stress can be reduced as much as possible.

It is critically important that the key people in the dyslexic person's life understand what causes stress for this individual. The following factors are keys to helping the dyslexic person overcome failure and develop adequate self-confidence. If the important people in the dyslexic's life can understand these critical issues, the effects of stress can be reduced to the level of being a nuisance instead of being a crippling condition.

Structure

The most critical skill dyslexic persons must develop is knowing how to maintain structure in their lives. The nature of dyslexia is for details to be out of order or out of sequence. Being dyslexic is not holding onto clear mental images of how parts go together in a certain order to produce a functional whole. Every moment of every day, the dyslexic person has to deal with mixed images, partial memory of details, confused sense of time passing, incomplete awareness of direction and where things are located, when it is time for the next important activity, how much money has been spent already, how much money is left to meet the budget before next payday, how many steps are yet to be done before the job is completed, and so forth. Persons who rank at Level 3 or lower on the severity scale have little difficulty learning how to stay organized. They learn early in life to use cues and reminders. They learn to cover their scrambled thinking well enough so that few outsiders ever suspect that this invisible problem exists. Persons at Level 4 or Level 5 cannot fully hide their trouble with structure, but they also manage to get by, although they face continual criticism and complaints about being "forgetful" and "scatter-brained." Level 6 and Level 7 dyslexics face lifelong struggles keeping their lives structured. Those who stay at Level 8 or Level 9 all their lives suffer tremendously from the stress of constant failure because their lives are so poorly ordered.

Until puberty has fully begun during the early teens, most dyslexics at all levels on the severity scale need help with structuring and organizing their lives. Preschool youngsters who later are found to be dyslexic are much more clumsy, poorly plugged into their world, and less able to manage themselves than are their peers who are developing normally. Dyslexia in early childhood creates problems with specific memory, and this places great stress upon the child as adults urge him or her to tell, describe, remember, and perform. "Jay, tell Grandma what we saw in the park yesterday," Mom says. Jay is stuck. He is partly blank. He remembers going to the park, but he does not have a full image of what went on there. "You know, Jay," mother says as she tries to show him off to Grandma. "We saw that great big brown animal with the big teeth!" Still Jay is partly blank and confused. "Dog?" he finally blurts out. "No, Jay, you know it wasn't a dog. Think hard now. Tell Grandma what animal we saw." If Jay is a sensitive child, he is already almost ready to panic. If Grandma joins this urging him to remember and tell her, he is suddenly under stress from two key people in his life. If Grandma should also add a bribe by saying: "I've got something nice in my purse for a little boy who can tell me what he saw in the park," the stress may become unbearable. Even before anyone has discovered that little Jay is dyslexic, he is living with the stress of failure.

Many little children like Jay are too sensitive to deal with this kind of early failure. They burst into tears as Mom and Grandma press for specific language structure the child cannot give. Jay's oral language processing is too loose to let him remember specific details in a given order. He needs help with his language structure. But instead of help he often receives criticism, even though it may come under the camouflage of loving adults pressing him too hard to remember. Time after time over a period of delicate years as the child's ego is formed, stress takes its toll in self-confidence. This kind of poor language structure in early childhood usually imprints lasting scars upon self-image and self-worth, especially if Jay has a sibling who blurts out answers for him or "shows him up" by being more successful.

Richard and Mary Masland have published an excellent anthology of studies of delayed language development in preschool children (Masland & Masland, 1988). Such researchers as Wilson and Risucci (1988); Keogh, Sears, and Royal (1988); Lundberg (1987); and Jansky (1988) are mapping language patterns that predict future learning problems for certain youngsters. These and other studies document the effects of the early language struggle and stress these children endure as they try to interact verbally with the world around them. Enormous frustration is an integral part of delayed language development, whether the child later is dyslexic or a "late bloomer."

Earlier chapters have made the important point that the label *dyslexia* should never be applied until a certain amount of evidence has been accumulated. It is usually not possible to determine dyslexia until the child reaches age 7½ or 8 years. Many youngsters who stumble over poor structure are late bloomers, not dyslexic. But whether the child is poorly organized because of a brain-based dysfunction or late maturity, the process of helping must be the same. The poorly organized child must have help with any task or situation that requires him or her to deal with structure.

Supervision Strategies

Perhaps the greatest problem adults face in working with dyslexic children is the youngsters' resistance toward being supervised. Yet these vulnerable youngsters cannot learn to cope with stress without supervision. This universal stubbornness in dyslexics is partly due to their different view of the world. They do not register the same impressions of events. They do not scan their world with the same degree of insight. They do not come away from experiences with the same quality of impressions. They do not look back with the same perspective. They do not judge time, dimension, distance, space, or reality the same way others do. They do not react to stimulus with a whole, fully integrated response, but they continually leave out some important ingredient that alters how they should have reacted. They tend to respond more slowly than others, which causes their understanding to be delayed. They have the tendency to "freeze" in unexpected situations, which looks very much like balking or stubbornly refusing to cooperate. They often do not know what to do in situations where others know automatically or quickly figure out the right response. If dyslexics are left alone to decide for themselves, they are out of step, in conflict, at cross purposes, and in danger as the fast-moving "traffic" of their society whizzes by on all sides. Being dyslexic in today's heavily loaded culture is like standing in the middle of a busy freeway. The risks for conflict are enormously high. Because of slow reaction time, faulty interpretation, incomplete recall, misunderstanding of signals, scrambled impressions, cluttered mental images, and uncertain body-in-space orientation, dyslexics must be supervised. They must have outside help to handle all the traffic on our culture's freeway. They cannot deal with their constant load of stress without guidance and a certain degree of supervision.

Parents of dyslexic children face the never-ending task of keeping the child's life structured so that as few loose ends as possible are faced each day. It is impossible for dyslexic children to be on time for meals, gather up necessary things for school, get dressed on schedule, remember a string of instructions, do a series of jobs that were told to the child that morning, keep everything picked up in their rooms, bring all of the outside things into the house or garage at night, take care of pets, and so forth. The memory patterns of dyslexic children simply cannot cope with the hundreds of facts and sequences that are part of normal living. These children must have supervision. Yet the supervisor must be kind, not aggressive. The supervisor must be helpful, not overly critical. The supervisor must be patient, not angry over delays. The supervisor must stay calm, not yell or lash out at the confused child. The supervisor must walk by the child's side as a guide, not push from the back as a prodder. Dyslexic children need supervision because they cannot see the next few steps clearly. It is much like someone peering into a dark corridor, wondering what is just ahead. Anyone would naturally pause before starting down a dark, unknown passageway. Dyslexics pause hundreds of times each day because the next moment is not clear. The supervisor must realize that this balking is not just because the child is being stubborn. It is because the child is afraid.

At those moments of hesitation, the dyslexic youngster faces a dark unknown. If the supervisor takes the time to shed enough light, then the child can move forward safely and confidently. If the supervisor shoves the indecisive child roughly or impatiently forward, the the dyslexic youngster feels panic and impending failure. The role of supervisor is that of guide, not of taskmaster. This child with faulty memory and incomplete perception will respond to a guiding hand that reassures that all is well. However, the dyslexic child will freeze, panic, and rebel the moment that stress is felt too keenly. Fear is the constant shadow of the dyslexic individual of whatever age. Fear of failure, fear of being incompetent, fear of being rejected, fear of being criticized, fear of humiliation, fear of being impotent when others can do it well, fear of losing loved ones or cherished relationships, fear of dying, fear of being "dumb," fear of not living up to the expectations of special persons in one's life. Such fear freezes the ability of the dyslexic child to move ahead on schedule.

This underlying aura of fear flavors every decision the child must make. The aftertaste of fear fills the emotions the way a bad smell fills a room. The haunting memory of other failures triggers faster heartbeat and physical constrictions that cause the chest to tighten, breathing to quicken, and blood pressure to soar. The frightened child is on guard, overly defensive, and on the verge of running away from the unknown. The dyslexic child under too much stress, without enough helpful supervision, wants to hide or escape. It is less painful to be scolded again for forgetting homework than to go through the agony of making another failing grade. It is easier to endure another reprimand for being lazy than it is to do one's best, when that best is not good enough for a critical adult.

Older dyslexics often are criticized for "not taking that good job," or subjected to comments such as, "Why did you quit your job? That's four jobs you've quit already this year!" What the critic does not realize is that the pain within the fearful dyslexic finally becomes too much to be endured. Dyslexics are never fully free from uncertainty. It taints their emotions the way garlic taints the breath. If the right kind of supervision is provided early enough, most dyslexics can learn to overcome this innate fear and develop strategies of coping with stress successfully.

Supervision can come in a variety of ways. Most dyslexics need a key person who is the main source of their supervision. With children, this will usually be one parent, usually mother. In single parent families, the parent is not always available to supervise and keep the child on schedule. Many dyslexic children turn to substitute parents for this form of help. In fact, most dyslexics find someone on whom they can depend for help. Adults often complain about the kinds of friends their children prefer. It is natural for fearful, apprehensive, or insecure youngsters to seek out companions who do not judge, criticize, or scold them. Dyslexics usually become attached to other dyslexics because no one else is patient enough. When two or three dyslexic individuals form a group, they are actually developing their own community or substitute family where they feel welcome and free from the stress of judgment. Why should dyslexic children want to associate with those who continually nag, criticize, judge, scold, and make them feel like failures? Bonding to a group of companions who accept dyslexic thinking as normal is part of the process of finding a source of help that gives without always taking away. Occasionally a dyslexic child finds supervisory companionship in an older brother or sister. Sometimes grandparents serve this important role, as do uncles and aunts. Sometimes the supervisor is a scout leader, a coach, a church leader, a teacher, a school custodian, a neighbor who operates a small business nearby. Many adults become the surrogate parents for dyslexic young people when they provide the patient, nonjudging guidance these youngsters need.

The most important kind of supervisory strategy is something the dyslexic can see. Few dyslexics can develop full mental images just by listening or doing abstract thinking. They must see some kind of outline, some kind of sketch, some kind of graph or chart or diagram, before concepts begin to make sense. Even when dyslexic persons are good listeners and glean most of their new information through listening, they still need to encode it some way in a visible pattern that can be seen, pondered, touched, and examined over a period of time. Early in the nurture of a poorly organized child, parents must begin to develop visible structure clues and guidelines.

Color Cues

Earlier chapters of this book have discussed the role of the right brain in learning new information. The right brain is the nonword brain. The right brain does not call things by name. It recognizes things by shape, size, color, form, texture, place, position, and so forth. Long before children are ready to read words or interpret alphabet letters or numerals, they can follow right-brain structure. Poorly organized children who later will be identified as having learning disability must have a lot of right-brain structure in their early years. Specific places in their room must be coded. If the child shows good perception of color, then the room should be color coded. For example, bright red would show where socks and underwear always go. Bright blue would show where pajamas go. Bright yellow would show where shoes always go. Bright green would show where books always go. The child's socks would have bright red marks. Pajamas would have a bright blue patch. Shoes would have bright yellow spots. Books would have bright green. Whatever the child is expected to organize and keep in place would be coded by visible color that would not be named by the left brain but would be recognized and matched by the right brain.

Shape Cues

Some children do not respond to color cues. For instance, from 3% to 7% of all boys are "color blind." If color is not feasible, other types of right-brain structure cues are possible. Some parents use geometric shapes as markers. Shoes go where the child sees a large square. Books go with the circle. Pajamas go with the triangle. Many families follow through by coding tools and equipment with right-brain cues. The child learns to match the color on the tool with the hook or drawer of the same color. It is much easier to guide a disorganized child through the chore of cleaning up his or her room, or putting tools back in the right place, if the supervisor uses right-brain cues: "Now, John let's find all of your red things. That's good. Now let's find all of the green things. Do you remember where green things go? Look for the green drawer (or hook). That's right. Now let's find all of your blue things." Or some creative children like to use animal cues. Shoes go in the bird drawer. Books all go on the elephant shelf. Pajamas always go with the kangaroo. Socks and underwear always go inside the dinosaur drawer. These kind of right-brain structure cues can reduce stress unbelievably in the lives of poorly organized children and their families. From the earliest experiences with organization, the child is trained to look for how things are alike and different, how certain things belong together in categories, how specific cues show the right place, and how to follow instructions. But the key is to give visible, right-brain guidelines for the poorly organized youngster. It is impossible for these uncertain children to work structure out for themselves.

Lists and Outlines

As soon as children can read even simple words, the supervisor should start using lists and outlines. Each task to be done is written or printed on a list. Each task is clearly numbered. If only one task is to be done later, it is written on a list. When two or three tasks are to be done that day, a list is prepared by the supervisor. The child learns where the list will always be. The supervisor does not change locations of the list. Once the child is told where his or her list will be each time, that place stays the same. When the supervisor says: "Jay, go look at your list," Jay does not have to wonder where it is.

Written lists remove nagging from the relationship between supervisor and child. When adults try to supervise orally, they inevitably end up in shouting matches with the disorganized, forgetful child. "Jay, I told you to feed the dog." "No, you didn't." "Yes, I did! You never listen to a word I say!" Verbal arguments over who said what are removed by posting a simple list:

1. Feed the dog.
2. Water the dog.
3. Wash your hands.

Supervisors of disorganized youngsters must be prepared for these youngsters' tendency to split hairs. Most adults make the mistake of underestimating the intelligence of a child who is loose and poorly organized. As was pointed out in earlier chapters, dyslexics are usually much brighter than average. They often do not score well on timed, standardized intelligence tests or standardized achievement tests, but in reality they are basically quite intelligent. Their intelligence is loose, poorly organized, and often beyond their reach in organized left-brain work. This underlying intelligence fosters a lot of splitting. Many supervisors of dyslexics become intensely frustrated by the tendency to quibble. Many dyslexics split hairs over tiny details that the busy adult did not think to mention. In giving instructions, the supervisor assumes that the child will use common sense in interpreting what was said. A simple statement, "Feed the dog," includes a lot of assumed material that the busy adult did not think necessary to say. But many dyslexics split as they interpret, especially if they would rather be doing something else. For example, the following dialogue is typical of the splitting that often occurs when supervisors take shortcuts:

Adult: Jay, don't forget to feed the dog this evening.

Jay: OK.

When the adult comes home from work at 5:30 p.m., the dog has not been fed.

Adult: Jay! I told you to feed the dog when you got home from school! You don't ever do anything I say!

Jay: No, you didn't.

Adult: I certainly did! This morning I told you to feed the dog when you got home from school! Don't tell me I didn't tell you!

Jay: That's not what you said. You said to feed the dog this evening. It's not evening yet. Evening starts when the sun goes down.

This kind of splitting goes on continually between dyslexics and supervisors. This is one of the hazards of giving instructions orally. This kind of arguing is greatly reduced and controlled when the supervisor takes time to make a specific visible list.

1. Feed the dog when you come home from school.

2. Check the dog's water.

3. Close the garage door so the dog can't get out.

Then the adult need only ask: "Jay, did you do everything on your list?" This places the responsibility back on Jay and avoids nagging and yelling over what was said that morning. If Jay has chosen not to look at the list, then he is responsible for the consequences. He cannot wiggle out of responsibility by splitting hairs over what was or was not said orally.

Memory Guides

As children move upward through the grades in school, they must learn to handle a multitude of memory tasks. Each new year introduces still more things to be remembered. Homework must come home along with necessary books and papers to do it. Next day, homework must be taken back and handed in to each teacher to receive a grade. Long-term assignments such as book reports, science projects, and term papers must be done on a schedule. Many youngsters do not go directly home from school. In fact, our society now includes several million "latchkey children" who are left alone from early in the morning until late afternoon by working parents. Millions of young people take music lessons, gymnastics training, and participate in sports after school. Teenagers work part-time before and after school. Many youngsters attend religion classes on certain evenings of the week. From kindergarten upward, life becomes increasingly complex for today's children and families. It is imperative that loose, poorly organized youngsters be taught how to keep their duties and obligations organized.

Calendar

Chapters 1 and 2 explained the poor sense of time and chronology that complicates life for most dyslexics. They do not have a built-in sense of time passing, of a sequence of events, or of how one event relates to a series of others. They must *see* time to deal with it successfully. This calls for early use of a personal calendar. As soon as children become involved with day-to-day activities, they must start seeing their days, weeks, and months represented on a calendar. Before they can read the names of days and months, they need right-brain symbols. Again, each day can be a certain bright color. On the blue day they take lunch money to school. On the red day they have a music lesson after school. On the green day they ride in the carpool to church for youth activities. On the yellow day they take gymnastics lessons. On the purple day they practice soccer. As soon as the child begins to work with letters, words, and numbers, these are added to the calendar. The adult supervisor takes a few minutes each day to go over the week's calendar with the child. This continual, consistent repetition begins to build a foundation for helping the youngster think in terms of time and how events are related. He or she begins to see how one event comes first, another comes next, another occurs later, and so forth. By the time the child has seen his or her life represented in this calendar form for several years, a lifelong organizational skill has been established.

Daily School Log

Today most students carry book bags. It is now fashionable for boys as well as girls to carry their things in bags. This provides an important way for the supervisor to help dyslexic youngsters stay organized. Each evening the adult guides the student in making a simple log (list) of everything that must go back to school the next day. Everything is included on the log. Nothing is assumed. The supervisor makes sure about pencils, tablets, art supplies, erasers, or whatever the student needs to do his or her work properly. Does the child need new supplies? Have any teachers told the class that certain things will be needed for upcoming assignments or projects? Does the student have all of his or her assignments finished? The supervisor and student go over the log together before bedtime. Then next morning another quick review of the log is done. The adult says: "John, take time to go over your log again. I don't want you to forget anything that needs to go back to school." If John protests that he does not have time, the supervisor reminds him that he is responsible. He is not to call Mom or Dad from school telling them that he left something important at home. Again, the log becomes the source of pressure. If the student decides to take shortcuts, then he or she must face the consequences. If it was on the log, then the log will be the final authority.

Dyslexics must live by lists and calendars all their lives. They have no choice but to encode their responsibilities in a visible form. They cannot handle the stress of responsibility just by memory. Early in their lives, they must develop habits of organizing their activities, responsibilities, and choices around some kind of calendar or visible list. Successful dyslexics carry pocket reminders everywhere they go. They develop ways of making quick notes of whatever they must remember. They keep lists of words they cannot spell but must write frequently. They keep lists of phone numbers, names of people they will see often, clues about finding locations, birthdays and anniversaries, and so forth. They must learn to keep track of money by developing a budget log of how much they have spent and how much is left. They carry small calendars showing long-range schedules such as coming holidays and vacation times. These are supervisory methods that are essential for dyslexics of all ages. The personal supervisor of childhood gradually changes to the written supervisor that reminds at a glance. If these kinds of organizational strategies are taught to dyslexics, they can become free from much of the stress and uncertainty that threaten them at every turn.

Becoming Independent

As dyslexics become older teens and young adults, they go one of four ways. Most dyslexics gradually replace Mom or Dad with a close friend, usually someone they are dating. As a special friendship or romantic relationship develops, most dyslexic teens become dependent upon this new important person. Girls often become new supervisors for dyslexic boys. Occasionally, a nondyslexic boy becomes supervisor for a dyslexic girl of whom he is fond. These relationships tend to become intensely emotional and usually are lopsided. The relationship actually becomes a parent-child situation with the supervisor taking the place of Mom or Dad. Although romance often is the basis for their relationship, the partners find themselves in conflict when one person gives advice and instructions while at the same time being the object of romantic affection. The dyslexic partner often resents the parental role of the other, but he or she cannot get along without this help. It is often highly stressful for the dyslexic partner to be so dependent upon the one he or she loves. Not many teens are mature enough to realize all of the elements in these complex relationships. The strong bonding that occurs in romantic partnerships is in conflict with the nurturing bond that exists between the parent and the child. When a dyslexic falls in love with a nondyslexic person, it is very difficult for them to work through the stress and frustrations that emerge from their unequal needs unless they are willing to receive counseling.

When dyslexics marry, they usually choose spouses who can fulfill the role of supervisor. The nondyslexic spouse keeps the budget, makes the lists, manages the money, takes care of all the family details, reminds the dyslexic spouse when and where to be, and so forth. The supervisory spouse writes all the letters, pays the bills, plans for gift giving and birthday celebrations, keeps the family on schedule for holidays, and stays in touch with important relatives. Again, the relationship is not equal. The nondyslexic adult must play two roles at once. He or she must be a marriage partner, with all that implies, as well as being the "parent" who makes the lists for the "child." Many solid, comfortable marriages develop between a dyslexic adult and a nondyslexic partner. But the dyslexic spouse must be able to turn over the organizational chores to the other without feeling threatened or diminished. And the supervising spouse must be able to accept this dual role without complaint or criticism. It can be done, but it is difficult. Most marriages that include a dyslexic spouse are marked by conflict, resentment, and misunderstanding. The fact remains that someone must be the organizer and manager of time and schedules. It is not always possible for this relationship to develop without continual stress disrupting the family.

Not all dyslexics are ready to become independent of parents or childhood supervisors when they become adults. In fact, many American families still have adult children living with parents long after they have finished high school. In most instances, this continuing dependent relationship occurs because the dyslexic child was not prepared over the years to become an independent adult someday. The steps in teaching visible structure described in this chapter usually were not taken during childhood and early adolescence. The level of fear was not reduced through careful teaching over a long period of time. In many families, it simply was easier for the adults to do all of the planning and make all of the decisions without doing the work of teaching the dyslexic child how. It requires enormous patience for parents to prepare a dyslexic child for adulthood. Dyslexic children are like all others in that they mature at different rates. Some mature quite early and are ready for relationships with romantic partners in their early teens. Others are not. Many dyslexics are also late developers, reaching their late teens with the physical maturity of young teens. Many dyslexic men are not yet shaving daily at age 21, nor have their voices fully changed until age 22. When their peers were dating and practicing romance in 10th grade, these late bloomers had no interest in such activity. As children, they were too immature to fit in with their classmates successfully in kindergarten and elementary school. As early teenagers, they were too immature to take part successfully in middle school and early high school. As young adults, they are several years behind schedule in being ready to live alone without supervision or live with a partner successfully. So these late blooming, dyslexic young adults continue to live with parents who do not know how to help them other than to provide safe shelter. This population of learning disabled young adults struggle to find jobs at which they can make an independent living. When they work, it is usually for minimum wage which does not provide enough net pay to support them separately. Our culture is struggling to help several million young adults who do not have the necessary skills to live alone, support themselves, make their own decisions, or develop a successful living arrangement with a mate or partner.

Some adult dyslexics live alone. They have managed to develop simple lifestyles in which they avoid anything that requires complicated planning. They seldom have many friends. They usually pay for everything in cash since they cannot handle the paperwork of banking. They tend to be isolated, self-contained, and alone. They live on the edge of boredom, and they are often intensely lonely, but they choose this life alone because they can manage it without complication. Their social lives are restricted to only a few activities: playing an occasional game of pool; going to the park on their days off; attending movies; eating simple meals at the same fast-food restaurants; watching a lot of television alone. They do not read, and they often do not have a telephone. Often they have chosen to be celibate. They are suspicious of strangers who show interest in them, and they avoid crowds as much as possible. Contact with family is carefully controlled and limited. If they attend religious services, it is to sit at the back so as not to call attention to themselves because they feel too illiterate to read from the Bible or follow the printed words in a hymnbook. These loners are sometimes mentally ill to some degree. The Menninger Foundation is documenting a correlation between dyslexia and certain forms of mental illness that emerge during the early teens but subside in the early twenties (Jernigan, 1985). Sometimes these loners develop enough courage to enroll in a course to upgrade literacy or job skills. But mostly they spend their lives off to themselves, attracting little attention and managing their meager resources in frugal ways. They do not view themselves as being worthy of anything better. They exist at borderline poverty levels, but they do not question that position in life. Early in their lives they came to believe that such a simple place in life was all they deserved or should expect. Few of these loners had much stimulation as children. Their own parents often were not well educated. Childhood for them was largely without emphasis upon learning. If these lone dyslexic adults ever thought about more education, they concluded that it would be beyond their ability. We have no idea how many intelligent, potentially creative dyslexics have fallen through the cracks where these lonely single adults find themselves in their late twenties and early thirties.

Since the early 1970s, more than 70 studies have been done of the learning patterns and levels of literacy among men and women in prison (Jordan, 1974, 1977, 1988b). A startling fact has emerged regarding learning disability among adjudicated delinquents and convicted felons. Three out of four (75%) of the adolescent and adult males serving time within our penal systems show major signs of dyslexia. The average level of literacy skills among this dyslexic prison population is below fourth grade. Virtually none of these males serving time were identified as being dyslexic during their school years. Many were evaluated for the first time as they entered the prison program. The shattering truth is that many dyslexic males in our culture forfeit their freedom through crime. There are many reasons for this tragic loss. A majority of these males come from backgrounds in which education was unimportant. In many cases, there was no stable parenting during the formative years. Many of them came from impoverished economic lives where basic needs were not met during childhood and adolescence. But the critical factor in their becoming involved with criminal activity was their lack of literacy skills. They could not compete with better-educated individuals in the job market. They did not have the personal skills to deal with marriage successfully. They could not handle the reading and writing requirements of our society in order to establish stable lives. They had no valuable parenting models to follow in their efforts to be fathers and husbands. They entered their teens or young adult years mostly illiterate, insecure, unstable, and unskilled. The question must be raised: How many of these men could have been saved had their dyslexic patterns been correctly identified and supervised when they were open to teaching and guidance? Our society has paid an enormous price in the loss of these young men who otherwise might have been guided toward productive lives.

Developing Self-Esteem

Personal success rests upon a foundation that must be established during childhood if a man or woman is to build a stable, productive life. Each person must have a positive self-image to believe that he or she is worthy of good things in life. Self-esteem must be strong enough to give the person sufficient courage to risk failure in order to find success. Self-image must be positive enough for us to like ourselves. What one thinks of self determines how hard each individual is able to press toward success. Low self-image is like a strong hand on the shoulder that drags the person back when opportunity beckons us to step forward. Low self-esteem whispers: "You can't do that! No use to try! You would only mess it up like you do everything else!" Negative self-image continually tells self: "You're too ugly. Nobody cares for you. You're a loser. No one is going to give you a chance. You might as well forget about success. It is not meant for you."

During the 30 years in which I have worked with the learning disabled population, I have posed a question to several thousand dyslexic persons of all ages. After we know each other well enough to be comfortable together, I ask: "When you step out of the shower and look at yourself in the mirror, what do you see?" My question is meant as a metaphor, of course, not a physical act of staring at one's unclothed body in the mirror. But after more than a quarter of a century of asking this question, I am still astonished by the almost universal fear dyslexics have of "looking at themselves in the mirror." Eight out of 10 to whom I have posed this question have given me this kind of reply: "I don't look at myself in a mirror," or, "I can't stand to look at myself in the mirror." Only a few have enough courage and positive self-esteem to face themselves squarely without flinching or avoiding eye contact with self.

Those of us who spend our lives with dyslexics see certain causes for low self-esteem in this intelligent population. These sensitive people grow up under the shadow of judgment and criticism. Their mistakes continue day after day, year after year. Their best intentions are usually tarnished by failure. Their goals and ambitions are not realized because they usually dream beyond the practical limits imposed by their brain-based limitations. Their plans continually fall through when they take shortcuts and try to ignore their perceptual boundaries. Their comprehension of family standards and cultural taboos is often incomplete or faulty. These sensitive young men and women are especially vulnerable to certain factors that are usually not that critical for nondyslexic peers.

Guilt

A majority of the dyslexic children, adolescents, and adults I have known during the past 30 years have suffered from unresolved guilt. Occasionally I have met dyslexic men or women who are so intensely guilt-ridden they have become neurotic. Usually the level of guilt is more a nuisance, like a low-level toothache that never quite goes away. This pervasive guilt comes from several sources, all of which stem from the dyslexic person's failure to live up to some goal proclaimed by society or family. Specific sources of guilt are seen in many dyslexics as they fail to cope effectively with our culture's expectations.

A dyslexic child's family need not be religiously active to instill the concepts of guilt and sin. Most parents and members of the extended family hold certain strong beliefs as to what is right or wrong. Sometimes this is expressed through racial bias that teaches a young child not to associate with certain groups. Often this is expressed through religious bias that forbids mixing with different religions. A majority of dyslexic children grow up hearing religious teachings that implant strong, vivid mental images of God's wrath or punishment of certain activities. Most children gradually work out their own interpretation of religious teaching as they begin to read for themselves and develop broader understanding of truth and religious doctrine. Dyslexics cannot do so for themselves. Few dyslexics can study the Bible for themselves to find out what Scripture actually says about specific issues. The built-in auditory misperception problem of dyslexia makes it even more difficult for them to remember accurately what they hear in sermons, church school lessons, and family discussions of religious issues. I have seldom met a dyslexic person who had accurate or fluent knowledge of what his or her religion truly teaches. This special population often lives at the level of superstition. They grow up with primitive, incomplete understanding of religious doctrine or scriptural truth. It does not matter whether the child is receiving instruction for Christian communion, Jewish bar mitzvah, or other forms of religious training. Dyslexic youth cannot go to the printed source materials themselves and find out what the Word of God or church history says. They must rely upon adults to interpret religious matters for them. This is especially true of dyslexic youngsters who attend private church schools where truth and morality are often interpreted in strictly fundamental ways. It is too easy for dyslexic misinterpretation to occur as issues of right and wrong are presented by adult leaders.

Shane is typical of so many dyslexic men I have known. I first met Shane when he was a child. At age 10 he was at Level 8 on the severity scale for dyslexia. It was impossible for him to read, spell, do math computation, or maintain central vision without a great deal of supervision. He grew up in a strongly religious home where Christianity was interpreted in a strictly fundamental way. When his dyslexic problems were identified, he was enrolled in a private school sponsored by a fundamental church where issues of right and wrong were spelled out in a rule book for the students. Shane could not read the rule book, nor could he read the Bible which was quoted throughout the day by his instructors. I saw him periodically through middle school and high school years. Then he disappeared. He unexpectedly reappeared one day at my office door, one of the most troubled and desperate young adults I have seen. His handsome face was consumed by grief. His athletic body was slouched and disheveled. This attractive young man in his early twenties fell into a chair in my office and began to sob his heart out. After half an hour of crying, he looked around my office where he had been many times. Finally he dried his tears and said: "It is always so peaceful here. I always feel so safe." Like many others through the years, Shane had "come home" to a sanctuary where he knew that he would not be judged or criticized.

I finally learned that Shane had attempted suicide a few days before that visit. It was his third suicide attempt since his 16th birthday. He hid his face in shame as he blurted out his story. He could not look me in the eye. He tried to tell me what was causing his deep grief, but he could not choke out the words. Finally I took his hand and held him as I said: "You are about to die from guilt, aren't you, Shane?" He clung to me and sobbed: "How did you know?" "You are feeling terrible guilt because you have sinned," I said. He put his head down and sobbed, but he nodded yes. "This is all about sex, isn't it, Shane?" I asked gently. Then it all came gushing out. For the next 3 hours I listened to his torrent of confession of guilt. What a miserable sinner he had always been! What a dirty hypocrite he had turned out to be! Now there was no hope of salvation because God could not love anyone as dirty as he. This litany of guilt went on and on until Shane was exhausted. Then I asked what his awful secret sin had been all those years. "I want to have sex with girls," he blurted out. "But that's a sin. The Bible says a man will go to Hell if he thinks about having sex with girls. But I can't help it. It gets so strong sometimes I jerk myself off. Then I want to die because that's a sin and God hates any man who does that to himself. I can't go on living like this. I'm so dirty and filthy. I can't do anything right. I've disappointed you and if my Mom had any idea, she would throw me out of her house."

When the storm was finally over and Shane was calm, we carefully reviewed his concepts of sin and evil, right and wrong. Like so many other dyslexic men I have known through the years, he had locked onto several misunderstandings of what his religion taught or meant regarding sexuality. This misperception had colored his entire life. His naturally strong sexual drive had overshadowed everything else, creating a strongly neurotic condition that made it impossible for him to function successfully in school or on a job. He could not date successfully because of his "terrible secret." He isolated himself from normal social life because of his belief that inwardly he was filthy for thinking certain things about girls. He began to drink heavily and take drugs because he could escape his haunting sense of guilt when he was stoned or drunk. He began staying up all night because he was afraid to go to sleep. While asleep, he frequently had erotic dreams he thought would doom him to Hell. He had tried many times to read the Bible, but he could not find the scriptural passages that deal with morality and sexuality. He had driven himself into the emotional corner of believing that he was vile as a man, filthy in his Creator's eyes, and unfit as a member of society. This extreme level of emotional suffering had gone on for several years.

Eventually I asked Shane the question: "When you step out of the shower and look at yourself in the mirror, what do you see?" His reaction was astonishing. "I have never looked at myself in a mirror!"

he exclaimed. "How do you shave?" I inquired. "I hold a towel over my face," he said. "I use an electric razor and I feel where it is on my face. If I have to see part of my face, I move the towel just a little. I have no idea what my face looks like. But I know I'm very ugly." I gazed in awe at this handsome young man who could easily be a fashion model. "What does your body look like?" I asked, referring to his athletic build and obviously good muscle tone. "I have no idea," he replied. "I work out and stay in shape, but I don't know what my body looks like. I can't look at myself. I am too filthy and ugly."

This story is an extreme example of guilt, of course. But most dyslexics harbor some kind of unresolved guilt that partly disables their ability to function well in society. Few dyslexic men or women I have known describe themselves realistically or accurately. Virtually all dyslexics I know put themselves down when they talk about physical appearance, attractiveness, level of appeal to others, and how righteous they might be. Those who listen to the secret stories of dyslexics usually hear confessions of sin, inadequacy, failure, and unworthiness. This underlying sense of guilt is like smog over the landscape of a beautiful city. The natural beauty of the person is at least partially masked by a darkish cloud that blots out his or her personal worth. After King David's tragic experience with Uriah and Bathsheba, he wrote the poignant words in Psalms 51: "My sin is ever before me." This is often true with those who are dyslexic. Their perceptions of right and wrong, adequacy and inadequacy, holiness and unholiness, being worthy and unworthy are often skewed and incomplete. They tend to enter their adult years carrying unresolved burdens of guilt that have never been discussed or fully examined with someone they can trust.

It is critically important that supervisors of dyslexic children take great care to make issues of religion, sin and righteousness, and morality fully clear. It requires much patient teaching and reteaching to help dyslexic listeners comprehend the full message without omitting essential elements that change the meaning. Whatever the dyslexic child comprehends, that is what he or she believes to be the truth. When overly sensitive youngsters like Shane misperceive such vital issues as normal sexuality, the misunderstanding sets into motion lifelong consequences that can disable the person emotionally and spiritually. This adds enormous stress to the already stressful life of growing up dyslexic.

Personal Appearance

Few of us would win the prize at a beauty contest. Most of us of whatever age must make the best of the physical endowments we inherit. How one's body is shaped, the characteristics of eyes and ears, the structure of one's face, the quality of one's teeth, all of these factors are part of one's self-image. The level of one's self-esteem is closely tied to personal appearance. This is especially critical for dyslexics. These sensitive persons must deal continually with the risk of failure and the stress of probably making a mistake within the next few minutes. If the body is not attractive, then it becomes all too easy to slip into the pit of low self-esteem that is so difficult to escape. Young people who are not dyslexic have trouble with poorly aligned teeth, slightly crossed eyes, severe acne, ears too large, being skinny or too fat, and so forth. Thoughtful parents do what they can to remedy these physical problems as children mature. If a dyslexic child also has physical problems that diminish appearance, then self-image suffers heavily in a culture that emphasizes good looks.

I remember many highly intelligent, overly sensitive dyslexics whose parents did not have the insight to recognize the importance of their child's physical appearance. For example, countless times over a 10-year period I had to calm Mark down when he became enraged over his "crooked teeth." This unusually handsome boy did have poorly aligned teeth that could have been corrected easily through orthodontal care. But his father saw no need to spend money for that kind of thing. The boy grew up watching his dad drive new Cadillacs and park expensive boat-and-trailer rigs in the driveway, but there was never any money for Mark's dental care. At age 36 this dyslexic man is still angry over his "ugliness" caused by his father's ignorance and stubbornness. It has colored all of Mark's self-image and self-esteem. His self-image is that his mouth is "ugly" and that his smile is offensive to others. In reality, he is a strikingly good-looking man, but his inner view of himself is the opposite. Lack of parental concern for this boy's physical appearance instilled a lifelong attitude of being "ugly" and unattractive. This low self-esteem made it much more difficult for teachers to reach Mark on an academic level.

Jill was always overweight and chubby, and she was also dyslexic. School performance was very difficult. Her learning disability was not identified until age 15. By then her parents had concluded that their daughter was "just fat and lazy." Discovering that she had a brain-based learning dysfunction did not change their attitude. During her critical teen years, Jill became obese, which fulfilled her parents' claim that she was just a "fat, lazy slob." In the 10 years I have known her, I have never seen Jill look anyone in the eye. When she talks with me or anyone else, her eyes look elsewhere. She looks at me frequently with rapid, darting glances to see if I am listening as she talks. But when her eyes contact mine, she blushes deeply and immediately turns her head. Her self-esteem is so low she cannot tolerate the normal interaction that comes with eye contact between friends. After working at a series of low-paying child-care jobs, Jill met a man who liked her and wanted to know her better. She was astonished that any man could be interested in her at all, given her obesity. As the friendship progressed, she joined a weight reduction club and eventually lost a hundred pounds. As her physical appearance improved, she began to use makeup attractively and dress in better fashion. But her self-image remains low. No matter how good Jill looks, she cannot make eye contact as she talks with friends. There are too many ghosts from the past, too many voices still criticizing her appearance, to let her believe that anyone could ever find her attractive or interesting.

It is of critical, lifelong importance that dyslexic children be encouraged to look their best and make the most of their attributes. The brain-based deficits that make life so complicated need the best possible packaging to allow dyslexic persons to overcome their limitations and enter the culture successfully. It is tragically false economy for families to save a few dollars during childhood years by not providing orthodontal care, acne treatment, or basically good grooming instruction. Self-esteem is already too easily fractured in these struggling learners. To face life with deficits in physical appearance in addition to the underlying cognitive deficits is too much for many of these fragile ego structures. Of all our children, dyslexics are the most urgently in need of support in developing strong self-image and positive self-esteem.

Chronic Failure

The most destructive factor for the self-esteem of dyslexics in our culture is chronic failure. To be dyslexic in the American culture is to risk failure at virtually every turn. This failure can be invisible moments when the memory "shorts out," but the dyslexic person recovers quickly enough so that no one else notices the loss. Inwardly, however, he or she feels the discordant twang of near failure. Failure can occur as the dyslexic starts to write. Suddenly the mental image is blank and the pencil will not begin its task of encoding. The fingers are stuck while the memory searches for the lost data. It can be a missing number, the spelling of a familiar word, the beginning letter of one's own name, or which direction to turn the pencil to form the needed written symbol. Failure can occur momentarily as the dyslexic person turns a corner and suddenly loses his or her body-in-space orientation. The mental image of north, south, east, or west vanishes.

The awareness of which is left or right disappears. The dyslexic freezes, not knowing at that moment which way to turn. Again, these invisible stumbling points may not be observed by others. But inwardly, the dyslexic has once again failed to carry out a normal procedure. Speaking is filled with hazards for dyslexics. The tongue may twist over a certain word or string of syllables, causing another "tongue twist" moment when the flow of articulation gets stuck. The word may be lost altogether, creating yet another moment of awkwardness when the speaker cannot continue his or her flow of speech. When dyslexia is below Level 5 on the severity scale, these chronic "blips" are usually managed well enough so that no one else notices or pays attention. But when dyslexic patterns are above Level 6 in severity, the moments of stumbling, reversing, or losing one's body in space become obvious and embarrassing. When dyslexia is above Level 7 in severity, the person is continually being corrected by others or scolded impatiently by tone of voice that implies if it does not say: "Why can't you ever get it right? How many times have you been told how to do it right?" Over the years, this chronic smog of failure engulfs the developing ego structure of the dyslexic person, blocking out the warmth of praise and admiration required for healthy self-esteem to develop.

I became painfully aware of the lifelong effect of chronic failure during a counseling session with Jay who was 19 years old. He had never been able to attend a full year of school because of intense school phobia. Chronic failure during his childhood, along with harsh scoldings and punishment from his father, had created a neurotic personality structure that was too fragile to cope with group participation. Three times he had erupted into a violent frenzy at school trying to defend himself. Three times he had been committed to mental health facilities for treatment of his "personality disorder." None of the mental health professionals recognized the severe dyslexic patterns in his language skills. I met Jay when he was 17, and he opened himself to me for the first time in his life. He trusted me to be gentle with his disabilities and not to criticize his weaknesses. He shared extraordinary poetry and song lyrics he had composed during his years of isolation from kids his own age. When he was 19, we began talking in depth about his secret thoughts regarding himself and his failure to relate to the outside world. At that time he was living alone in an apartment that was funded through a program for handicapped adults. I asked Jay if he ever visited places where he could meet young adults his own age. He said that he had gone to a few singles bars, and occasionally he had gone to church. But it did not work, and he had decided never to try it again. "Why not?" I asked. Without hesitation he made one of the most profound statements I have ever heard a dyslexic person say: "Because I don't have any stories to tell," he said.

Those eight simple words gave me a tremendously important piece to add to the puzzle of dyslexia. After working with this special population for 25 years, I finally understood a major reason why self-esteem is so difficult for them to develop. Chronic failure makes it very difficult, often impossible, for these strugglers to develop good stories to tell. I had not thought about that before. What do we all do when we get together? What happens at Sunday school or at the barber shop or when friends meet in the supermarket? What takes place when neighbors meet over the back fence or in the hallway or in the parking lot? What goes on continually where we work and when we travel? What is happening in those moments before the worship service starts or the concert begins? We tell stories. All kinds of stories. Most of our stories are good. We chat on and on about the little things that have happened, what our children are doing, the victories we have achieved, the problems we have solved. We gossip about people we know. We complain about our jobs or we wish things were better where we spend our days. We confide little things about our lives. Sometimes we tell difficult stories about sorrow or misfortune. But we spend a great deal of our social time telling stories.

Severely dyslexic persons, and even many moderately dyslexic individuals, often do not have good stories to tell. Jay explained it so clearly: "Sure I have stories to tell. But who wants to hear my stories about getting kicked out of school, or being committed to the mental hospital three times, or being put on drugs to make me calm, or how my dad yelled and cussed me out? What kind of girl wants to go out with a guy who tells stories like that? And you know the weird sex fantasies I have a lot. I sure can't tell those stories to decent people. And nobody wants to hear my stories about being afraid all the time and being paranoid about strangers. I sure don't have any good stories to tell about school. Who wants to spend an evening listening to my stories about flunking third grade and being kicked out of elementary school? You're the only person I ever met who will even listen to my stories and not think I'm crazy."

Jay's case is extreme, of course, yet his chronic failures at school, at home, and in society are a mirror of what most dyslexics experience to some degree. Yet it need not be this way. Dyslexic children who are blessed with patient, observant parents do develop good stories to tell. Dyslexic students who are fortunate enough to spend years with patient, flexible teachers develop anthologies of good stories to tell about ways in which they succeeded within the school environment. They did not make top grades, but they were given opportunities to earn praise, which is what good story telling is all about. Dyslexics who have thoughtful, caring coaches develop many good stories to tell through athletic success and sports achievement. Dyslexics with strong right-brain talent for drawing, painting, crafts, and tool handling emerge into their teens and early twenties with good stories to tell and show. Dyslexics who meet caring romance partners who accept left-brain limitations without rejection have many good stories to tell of love and warm friendship. Good scout leaders give many struggling boys and girls good stories to tell by helping them achieve rank and complete merit badge goals. Caring 4-H Club leaders often guide dyslexics to national championships in livestock and agricultural projects, and these are great stories to tell the rest of one's life. Patient bosses on the job who are not irritated by needing to repeat instructions until the dyslexic employee knows the task contribute good stories through job success. The key to developing good stories to tell is patient leadership. When supervisors of dyslexics are patient, thoughtful, and careful to make things clear, dyslexics like Jay do indeed develop a repertoire of good stories to tell.

Positive self-image develops in dyslexics through little "baby steps" over a period of time. Those who are not handicapped by left-brained limitations judge success by long strides forward. Dyslexics gain success a little at a time. Dyslexic children who are fortunate enough to have compassionate, observant parents from the beginning make progress in small steps all of their lives because self-esteem was continually supported and nurtured. Language gaps are gently supplemented, not criticized. Directional confusion becomes part of a funny family game as everyone thinks of ways to help the dyslexic remember left and right, or north/south, east/west. All kinds of memory tricks are developed through rhymes and simple ways to keep things straight. Dyslexia is handled with a good sense of humor, not with scoldings and punishment when awkwardness or forgetfulness occurs. Every "baby step" of progress is praised, the way star pupils are praised for outstanding achievement. Moments of fear that cause the child to freeze are treated thoughtfully, not with criticism. Impulsiveness or lapses of good judgment are absorbed by the family as the child is guided once more through the family standards of right and wrong. The tongue twisters and malapropisms that all dyslexics create are treated with delight, as the child makes a major contribution to the family's fun and joy. Parents and relatives look for the natural bent, the underlying talents, and help the child grow in those unique areas, even though standard left-brain skills remain difficult. Over a period of years, all of these "baby steps" carry the child through adolescence and finally into adulthood with a healthy ego structure, strong self-image, and positive self-esteem. This fortunate dyslexic person enjoys looking into the mirror because the image looking back is good and worthy of praise. The dyslexic who has good stories to tell is strong, intelligent, interesting, and alive with hope. But the stories come slowly over time. It is incredibly difficult for a dyslexic child to become an adult with good stories to tell unless there has been long-term support from a parent figure who knew how to reinforce that child's bent, not criticize for deficits. By the time I met Jay, it was too late. I shall always wonder what eternal difference it could have made had I met him and his parents when he was a child. Perhaps those bewildered adult supervisors could have learned how to deal with his needs more positively. If that highly sensitive boy had learned a few good stories to tell along the way, his adult self-esteem could have been salvaged and restored.

6

Helping Dyslexics Develop Social Skills and Independence

Most of the attention our society has paid to dyslexia has been toward the academic problems this disability presents. Academic dyslexia is indeed a massive issue, as we have seen in earlier chapters. Being dyslexic within our educational arena is to suffer chronic failure, humiliation, and frustration. As we have discussed, it is virtually impossible for a poorly educated dyslexic person to find success as an adult if job skills are too meager to allow good employment. No one would claim that academic dyslexia is unimportant or trivial. However, an equally vital face of dyslexia must also be recognized and treated if learning disabled persons are to succeed in their adult years. The costly, often devastating problem of socialization disorders among dyslexics is beginning to be recognized in our society (Duane, 1987; Osman, 1986; Silver, 1985). Developing social skills presents the same degree of struggle, frustration, isolation, and rejection encountered by dyslexic persons during their academic years. But socialization is much more personal. The term *socialization disorder* refers to a person's inability to fit into society successfully; read social signals correctly; respond to peers and associates appropriately; participate gracefully in the "tribal dance" of group living; develop effective relationships with partners, spouses, or loved ones; and so forth. In other words, being socially disabled means that a person stumbles through relationships the way dyslexic students stumble through the educational process. Social disability produces the same kinds of awkwardness in dealing with life that academic dyslexia produces in dealing with literacy skills. In viewing the life of a dyslexic person, we would probably conclude that if we had to choose between success in school or success in life, it would ultimately be more important for one to be socially successful. It is possible for an illiterate person to earn a living and be a contributing member to family and society. It is virtually impossible for a socially disabled person to establish and maintain a successful life once he or she has passed beyond the shelter of the school years.

Social disability is a heartbreaking pattern for those who must live with such a person. A socially disabled person is oblivious to the normal niceties that must be followed if one is to love and be loved. Dyslexics with socialization disorders cannot read the sometimes subtle signals that tell us how to deal with others. These persons do not see boundary markers that say: "Not just now. Give me some space." Socially disabled dyslexics are basically self-centered in that their major concern is for themselves. They do not have the sensitivity to realize when they are being too overbearing or too shrill or too demanding. They are too socially unaware to recognize when their own behavior has offended someone else or when their habits are embarrassing. They do not plug into the normal give-and-take that must occur in any successful relationship. They often display deep stubbornness that makes them impossible to influence, even when they are wrong and must change their ways. They often have poor manners that grate on the nerves of those who must share their space. They do not see how their decisions can be a problem to others, even when they are impulsive spenders or waste precious resources on trivial or immature things. They cannot understand constructive criticism. They tend to be overly sensitive and too easily offended when anyone suggests that they need to change. They do not follow through on plans, they do not see how their poor punctuality affects coworkers, and they cannot understand why they are unpopular on the job. They usually keep moving from job to job, not learning essential lessons from their mistakes. Married dyslexics who are socially disabled are usually insensitive to the needs of the spouse or children. Even though these adults may be affectionate and even good lovers, the overall business of building a marriage or rearing children over a period of years is often beyond their understanding. Most socially disabled dyslexics have "tunnel vision," seeing only a few issues clearly and not comprehending other important issues that also must be considered. As spouses they tend to be self-centered and blind to specific needs in loved ones. As parents they tend to be overly demanding and narrow in how they discipline. As workers on the job, they tend to be stubborn and inflexible when it comes to following instructions. As citizens they are generally uninformed on issues that affect society. Socially disabled teenagers tend to grow into strongly opinionated adults who harp on the same few issues, over and over and over. As they leave their twenties and move on toward middle age, they settle into narrow, shallow life-styles that become set in concrete. This means that any spouse or companion must do most of the adapting and changing as time goes by. Socially disabled dyslexics are often somewhat paranoid, never fully trusting anyone but themselves. They frequently flare into angry confrontations when their points of view are challenged or criticized. To emerge into one's adult years as a socially disordered person is costly to everyone involved in that person's life. Yet little attention has been paid to this cultural problem.

Is it possible to guide dyslexic children in such a way that they will not become socially disabled? As a point of reference, we need to look at a developmental pattern I have studied closely for 30 years. By participating in the lives of several thousand dyslexics from childhood into adulthood, I have discovered a pattern (Jordan, 1977, 1988b). If a child's dyslexic patterns are identified by age 7, and if good remedial teaching and home guidance are started at that point, 85% of those children can be taught to achieve academic success. At the same time, they can be taught to relate successfully with their world and thus not become socially disabled. This rate of success depends upon cooperation between home and school.

If dyslexic patterns are not identified until age 9, with remedial and guidance techniques not begun until that age, there is approximately a 70% chance for successful remediation. We lose 30% of our dyslexic population by waiting that long. If dyslexia is not identified and treated by school and home until teen years, only 5% of these older youngsters can be fully remediated. If dyslexia is not identified until early adult years, only a few individuals can be changed by that time. The point is that early identification and treatment can change the academic and social patterns that characterize dyslexia. As time goes by, it becomes increasingly difficult. Each passing year of academic failure and social struggle makes it less possible for deeply embedded patterns to be modified. The older the person, the longer he or she has lived in a climate of failure, conflict, and low self-esteem. Dyslexics can and often do reach a point of no return.

Profile of Social Disability Among Dyslexics

The pattern we call socialization disorder is composed of specific ingredients, all of which interact like the roots of a tree to support the complex structure of this disability. By looking at each ingredient separately, we can see how this personality style develops. This also gives us clues in helping the dyslexic person change habits and grow a different way.

Research by Duane (1987), Osman (1986), Blanchard and Mannarino (1978), Hippchen (1978), Wacker (1975), and others has produced the designation *Right Hemi Syndrome.* This describes a certain segment of the learning disabled population who have specific lesions within the right brain. Teenagers and young adults identified as having Right Hemi Syndrome display a certain type of irregular behavior: poor socialization, inability to keep personal relationships going, inability to lead within their peer groups, inability to interpret feedback signals from others, usually poor academic performance, difficulty finding employment, difficulty holding a job within their field of preparation, and so forth. This special population includes many dyslexics. Many also show major symptoms of Attention Deficit Disorder (ADD). They are difficult people in all types of relationships. Their thinking is largely dyslogical. They tend to be stubborn and narrow-minded. They continually alienate others through hostile or overly aggressive behavior. The following characteristics are usually seen in the lives of these socially disabled persons.

Self-Centeredness

The taproot of social disability is self-centeredness. This central problem supports the rest of the structure. Extreme self-centeredness is described in psychiatric terms as narcissism. In ancient mythology, Narcissus was a handsome young man who could not take his eyes or thoughts off himself. He spent long hours gazing at his reflection in pools and mirrors. He lost all contact with the outside world as he gazed at himself, loved himself, groomed himself, and thought only of himself. As the ancient myth goes, he eventually disappeared inside himself and was transformed into a lovely flower that looked at itself all day at the side of a pool. In modern terms, a truly narcissistic person would be mentally ill, incapable of normal emotional interaction with others. Dyslexics who are socially disabled are not mentally ill, except in isolated cases when true mental illness does emerge. But the socially disabled person is self-centered and thinks mostly of self. The primary concern of such a person is: "What do I get out of this situation? What is here for me? What can my friends and family do for me? What can I get for myself out of this new job? What does my roommate owe me for all I've done?"

This type of thinking dominates the waking hours of most socially disabled dyslexics. They simply do not see the needs of others. When they occasionally recognize that someone else has a need, the tendency is to do something impulsive for that person at the moment, then get back to the business of satisfying self. It is impossible for the socially disabled person to keep his or her attention focused very long on others.

Joe is a striking example of this socially disabled dyslexic self-centeredness. I met him when he was 9 years old, so frustrated in an elementary school classroom that he was having tantrums and disrupting everything the teacher tried to do. We formed an immediate bond, because I was the first adult ever to give this frustrated child the kind of attention he was starved to find. He loved me intensely in his self-centered way. As his guide and counselor, I was able to absorb his self-centeredness so that he felt great joy when we were together. His family could not help me with Joe's dyslexic tendencies. Their deeply embedded family style was that of confrontation. The relationship between mother and father was based upon competition to see which adult could outsmart and outwit the other. This often fierce rivalry was absorbed by the children who carried out this competitive spirit between each other. The family environment was that of finding fault with one another, seeking ways to dominate one another, never failing to remind one another of past mistakes, and making constant predictions of failure or family shame brought on by one another. Joe came into this arena unable to cope with such competition. To survive, he had to become a little gladiator, slashing his opponents as they slashed him. Being dyslexic in that intelligent but combative family was an excruciating condition for such a sensitive, perceptually limited child.

Many of us who work with dyslexics realize a critically important fact: If a dyslexic person can find two sources of positive support, then he or she can change from being socially disabled toward being an outgoing, socially successful person. If the home cannot give such support, but the child can receive that support at school and from some other important source, the negative influence of home can be overcome. If school cannot provide positive support, but the dyslexic child can find it both at home and from another important source, then the child can overcome the negative influences of the classroom. Joe was isolated from positive change both at home and at school. The stubbornness and self-centeredness of his parents kept them from agreeing upon the best school placement where his academic needs could be met. If one parent agreed, the other disagreed as part of their competitive pattern.

Joe went through school in a program that matched his home life in competition, criticism for failure, and lack of support for positive self-esteem. At home he was regarded by parents and siblings as a problem child and an embarrassment to the family. At school he was treated as a "lazy" boy who just would not try. His relationship with me was the only warm, accepting, positive oasis in his life, but it was not enough to prevent him from becoming socially disabled. To survive, he had to be self-centered. To be thoughtful of others at home or school was to open himself up to criticism and ridicule.

In his teens, Joe wrote many pages of poetry. The spelling was dyslexic and the language skills were primitive, but the poetry was warm and often beautiful. However, it was self-centered material. He was madly in love with many girls and young women, but in a self-centered way. It was impossible for him to understand when I explained the give-and-take required in love. He developed the habit of buying each new girl friend a single rose, which he presented over a candlelight dinner at a luxurious restaurant. At first each girl was overwhelmed and delighted. But within a few days or weeks, Joe would be telling me about how still another girl had rejected him for "some jerk not nearly as smart as I am." I would read a series of new poems he had composed, dyslexic spelling and all, which he sent to the former girlfriend, reminding her of what she had forfeited by refusing his love. It was impossible to make a dent in Joe's narcissistic patterns. He simply could not comprehend what I said about turning his attention from himself to others. "But I am one of the most thoughtful guys in town!" he would yell at me. "What do you mean, I am self-centered? I buy them roses. I take them to the nicest places to eat. I treat them like royalty!" "Yes, you do," I would say. "But why do you do all these things?" "So they will like me!" he would reply. He could not see his self-centeredness in all of those relationships.

Joe's social disabilities finally came to a peak in something he did one day. He brought me a set of photographs he had taken. Later I realized that he had shot three roles of film in that project. As he proudly watched me look through the stack of pictures, he kept asking: "How do you like my photography? Don't you think I'm good with a camera?" I was astonished as I kept turning to the next picture. Every shot was of Joe himself. He had used three rolls of film to photograph himself. By setting the timer, he could settle into a new pose, then the camera would snap yet another picture of himself. Joe had brought me 108 snapshots he had taken of himself, and he could not comprehend why I was not delighted. He simply could not see the point of my question when I asked: "Joe, why did you take pictures of yourself?

Why not take pictures of others?" He slammed out of my office in a tantrum yelling, "There you go, criticizing me again!" After his first year of college, Joe drove on a vacation trip with a friend. When he returned, he showed me a lot of good snapshots of his trip. I soon realized that every picture was one of Joe. "Where is your friend?" I asked. "I don't see him in any of the pictures." "Oh, I threw away all the pictures he was in," Joe said with a shrug.

Socially disabled persons who are also dyslexic do not always take pictures of themselves, of course, but their lives are centered upon themselves. They are rarely aware that this is so. In fact, most socially disabled persons I have known think of themselves as thoughtful, considerate, generous people. The blind spot is that they cannot see why they give gifts, do courteous things, remember birthdays, and so forth. Everything they do is designed to get something back in return. Their generosity is a means of receiving praise and satisfaction for themselves. They do not see real need in others. If they do, they immediately turn another person's need back toward themselves. If a socially disabled person sees a friend crying, for example, he or she may take the friend into a warm embrace. But instead of listening to the friend's need, the socially disabled person turns it back on self. "I know how you feel," Joe would say. "Boy, have I cried a lot myself. Why, last week I cried when a girl broke up with me. You know, there sure are a lot of immature girls in this town. They just aren't mature enough to appreciate a guy like me. Yeah, I've cried a lot myself. My mom and dad make me cry a lot, the way they criticize me all the time. You ought to be at my house and hear them yell all the time." By this time the friend with the problem has pulled away from Joe's embrace. The reality soon becomes clear that he is not really interested in the friend's problems. All he can think about is himself. And Joe faces yet another situation in which he is pushed away by someone who needed more than he could give.

Self-centeredness is common in children. In fact, one of the earliest habits children must learn is how to share their playthings in a group. One of the first social milestones during early childhood is learning how to share, not hold things back for oneself. Teachers and parents are delighted when youngsters learn this important social lesson of looking beyond themselves with playmates. The dyslexic child often has much difficulty learning this important social skill, but it can be taught if adults begin soon enough. As we have seen earlier in this chapter, self-centeredness can be turned around along with overcoming reversed letters and scrambled sequence if it is addressed soon enough. It is critically important that dyslexic children have models at home and at school of caring, sharing, thoughtfulness, and consideration of others. It is impossible for adults to demonstrate concern for others if they themselves are self-centered. Children like Joe must have at least two sources of this instruction if these deep-seated tendencies are to be altered. They must see models of unselfish behavior day after day. Over a period of years they must see the consequences of sharing and caring for others. It is true that many adults never learn how to give freely with no strings attached to their gifts of affection. But children like Joe must have several years of clear demonstration of unselfish affection if they are to change their self-centered bent. It can be done, if the effort does not come too late. Social disability can be avoided if the child has at least two strong sources of guidance and example in how not to be self-centered. This basic tendency can at least be modified enough to teach the child how to be graceful socially when it comes to noticing others and paying attention to their needs and interests.

Learning not to be self-centered involves certain basic concepts. It is a matter of teaching the dyslexic child how to read body language and emotional signs. This requires the same kind of careful coaching that goes into teaching phonics and reading when a child cannot "hear" the sounds in words. As dyslexics learn literacy skills, they can also master social awareness skills, if the instruction begins soon enough before habits and attitudes are set too deeply to be changed.

Noticing Others. Self-centeredness is constantly looking at self and paying attention to self. Social awareness is looking at others and paying attention to others. The first step is to change the point of focus, away from self to someone else. Over a period of time, the dyslexic child is taught what to do when he or she comes into a room. Adults explain: "Don't wonder 'What will everyone think about me?' That is a self-centered thought. Instead, look at each other person and speak to them. Look for signs that tell how they are. Is Mary happy this morning? How can you tell? Does her face show it? Do her clothes show it? Is Robert unhappy this morning? How can you tell? How does his face show it? How might his clothes show it? Is Mrs. Jordan happy today? Does she feel well this morning after her cold last week? How can you tell? Why don't you ask her if she feels better today? Did Jason have fun over the weekend with his dad? How can you tell? Listen to what Jason is saying. Is he telling happy stories about what he did with his dad? Or is he not talking about it at all? Look at Janice, the new girl in the class. Has she been crying this morning? How can you tell? Do her eyes look sad? Is there something nice you can say to let her know you are glad she is in your class? Remember how Robert is always losing his things? How can you tell if he has his pencil ready for class? Can you help him look for his pencil before the teacher asks him about it?"

These are the kinds of "baby steps" parents and teachers must take to help dyslexic children learn how to turn their attention away from themselves. Some homes and classrooms have a natural climate of thoughtfulness where children are immersed in an environment of caring and thoughtful attention to others. Some children are sensitive enough to follow these kinds of examples and learn to behave that way themselves. Others must be guided step by step, the way they must learn the multiplication tables. Socially disabled dyslexics come from homes and classrooms where this kind of specific, long-range thoughtfulness is not presented and taught. It takes many years of careful nurture with this kind of daily practice at noticing others before the natural bent toward self-centeredness is changed in the dyslexic person.

Reaching Out to Others. Through the past quarter century I have worked individually with more than 10,000 dyslexics of all ages. I have observed that one of the most difficult skills for them to learn is how to reach out to others. Most dyslexics must exert a great deal of conscious effort just to get through each day successfully. During their academic years, their energies must go into doing their best in difficult studies, keeping up with volumes of homework, dealing with the emotions of flunking tests and making low grades, absorbing criticism without being too badly hurt, and so forth. It is very hard for these strugglers to have enough emotional energy left over for others. But they must learn to do so to some degree. Again, they must see the model of reaching out before they can claim it for themselves. From their early years, dyslexic children must see this social skill demonstrated. Many families have a grouchy attitude toward helping others, and this is quickly absorbed by children. If parents complain about having to be generous, then children will have trouble being generous.

The lesson of reaching out to others was vividly implanted in my young mind at the age of 7 by a single action by my father. I have only a few clear memories of my father. He was stricken with cancer about the time I started to school, and this was toward the end of the Great Depression. Like so many other men and women of the late 1930s, my parents were out of work, and our family faced the terror of no income with three children to feed. My father's medical needs were supplied by the Veteran's Administration, but he had to live at a veteran's hospital to receive treatment for his malignancy. My mother and we three children moved into a very humble apartment that faced the alley in an impoverished neighborhood. My mother was trying to make ends meet on a total income of $24.00 per month. I vividly recall that day when my father came home for a brief visit on furlough from the hospital. We were in the tiny back yard near the alley enjoying this rare family time together when a shabbily dressed, very dirty man came along and asked for something to eat. As a 7-year-old, I had only a primitive notion of how scarce food was for our family, but I knew that we had to be very careful. There were no treats and no extra helpings. I knew things were bad and that my mother cried a lot. As the shabby man stood there asking for food, I saw my mother shake her head. Later I would realize how little she had for her own, let alone anything to share. But I was suddenly drawn to my father's face. He smiled at the stranger and asked him to sit down and rest. Then he turned to my mother and said: "Could you fix one of your egg sandwiches for this good man?" My mother's egg sandwiches were among the wonders of the world when I was 7 years old. It was a very special treat when I got to have one of her wonderful creations with a fried egg, a slice of cheese, and toasted bread. I vividly remember that scene as my dad rubbed the pain in his amputated leg, chatted with the stranger who had no place to go and nothing to eat, and showed me what it meant to reach out to someone beyond ourselves. I have never forgotten the gratitude as that stranger thanked my mother for her gift. An egg sandwich never brought more joy than hers did that day. As I have reflected on that scene so many times, I have realized what my father gave me that day when I was 7. He demonstrated what it means to reach out to others instead of feeling sorry for ourselves. That experience set into motion a lifelong pattern I have followed to this day.

Dyslexic children find it hard to reach out to others, but they can learn to do so if they see the model and learn the skill. The crippling limitation of being socially disabled is not having the ability to reach beyond oneself, except for selfish purposes. This deeply important social skill can be taught if we do not wait too long. If reaching out to others is demonstrated along with phonics, spelling, and math practice, the child can learn what it means to attend to the world beyond self. The child is taught to notice what others need. "Look at Mark. Why is he frustrated? Is there something you can do to help him find his eraser? Look at Sue. She can't get her pencil to draw that circle. Can you help her do it so she can finish her picture? Look at Joe. He can't see his math book under his jacket. Can you help him find it? Look at Mrs. Jordan. She dropped part of the math papers by her desk. Can you help her pick them up? Look at Mr. Jones, the custodian. He can't get all of his stuff through the door. Can you help him by holding the door open?" These small steps in reaching out to others soon turn the self-centered bent another way. The child learns that reaching out to others is its own reward. Helping someone in need brings its own burst of joy. The child does not need something in return. The act of being generous is a social skill, part of the "tribal dance" one needs to learn. Dyslexic children can learn this skill of reaching beyond self, even when their own resources are exhausted, if this modeling is begun soon enough. It must be regarded by adults as being as important as learning the ABCs.

Self-Pity

One of the most unattractive ingredients of social disability is self-pity. The "poor little me" syndrome is a major reason why socially disabled persons are unattractive. Of course, many who are not dyslexic also bog down in the swamp of self-pity. At times it feels good for any of us to have a pity-party. But the wholesome person will soon laugh and get back to the business of being mature. It is very easy for a dyslexic child to develop self-pity. "Nobody else has to do this much work. Why do I have to work so hard all the time? Gene makes good grades and he doesn't have to work all the time! How come my brother gets to ride his bike and I have to finish this homework? How come I don't ever get to play? I just have to work all the time! It's not fair! How come I have some old learning disability? I didn't ask to be born this way!"

All of this is true, of course. It is not fair to be born dyslexic. It is definitely not fair for one's siblings to get to play when the dyslexic child has to keep on with unfinished work. It is not fair to have to go to tutors and special classes or go to summer school and never get to play. It is definitely not fair never to have one's papers up on the bulletin board with gold stars. It is not fair never to make top grades when you know that you studied harder than the star of the class. It is not fair when adults say: "If you just tried harder! I know you can do it. You just won't try!" It is not fair to be smarter than your friend, yet he can read better and make better grades. It is not fair always to lose your words and get tangled up trying to tell stories and look dumb every time you answer in class. It is not fair never being able to finish a test first or never getting all of your work done but having to take it home. It's just not fair!

The antidote for self-pity is a good sense of humor. This is not easy for dyslexics to learn. How do you laugh about making poor grades? Where is the funny part of being "dumb" all the time? What is there to laugh about when you get lost turning corners and can't remember where you leave things? What's so funny about not being able to spell your own name? Where is the humor in getting things backwards or reading "Altus" when the sign said *Tulsa*?

Wise parents and teachers are able to help the student smile instead of lapse into self-pity. OK, so it's not very funny when all of these dyslexic things happen. But let's see how we can make the best of it. It helps to start with the really funny things that come along. For example, most dyslexics create marvelous tongue twisters that can be a lot of fun for the family. Families of dyslexics can actually be proud of certain verbal slips that turn into famous family sayings. One day Keith was explaining why he wanted to be alone for a while. "I just need to be synonymous," he said. And his family had a wonderful new way of talking about privacy. There was no criticism or embarrassment. There was praise and good humor over this rich contribution to the family vocabulary. One day Judy said that she had three "sliver dimes" in her coin collection, and her family suddenly had a new Judyism. Ever after that, they all looked for "slivers" when they counted their change. Alex became her "daddy's little gril" when she got her letters backwards, and that grew into her dad's tenderest term of endearment for his precious daughter. I knew that Stan had outgrown his self-pity when he brought me a wooden statue he had carved and painted so carefully. "This is my dyslexic sheriff," he explained with a smile. He showed me the word he had carved below the sheriff's foot: WARD. "That's dyslexia for DRAW," he laughed. One day Chris left his mom a note: "My book is no my bed." From then on, the family had a richly funny phrase. When anything was lost, they always said: "Look no the bed."

These are the kinds of "baby steps" we take in disarming the trigger of self-pity and turning it another way. But we have to begin this journey away from self-pity early, before the concrete hardens into inflexibility. I have seen many dyslexics reach their adult years without a sense of humor, and they are beyond the reach of others who would like to help them turn themselves loose. The ongoing pity-party is the habit of blaming others instead of taking responsibility for oneself. To feel sorry for oneself is to say: "It is not my fault." The pity-party point of view makes excuses for self and places the blame on others. "I inherited this problem from my dad, so it's his fault I'm dyslexic." "I had lousy teachers who didn't like me, so I never learned to read." "My math teacher was too lazy to do her job, so I never learned my times facts." "They didn't like me in junior high school, so I dropped out when I got old enough." "My boss worked me too hard, so I just quit. I won't work anyplace I'm not treated with respect." "My parents are partial to my older brother. That's why he drives a new car and I have this old junker." "Those cops are sneaky. That's why I have five traffic tickets." This litany of self-pity goes on and on until the person finds himself or herself in the position of being a loser. It is always the fault of others. If dyslexic children are not taught how to take responsibility and laugh at their mistakes, they tend to settle slowly into the swamp of self-pity. As years go by, they become encased in this attitude that is offensive to others and degrading to themselves. It need not turn out this way for most dyslexics, if children are taught to avoid self-pity along with avoiding reversals and other dyslexic traps.

Stubbornness

Socially disabled persons are usually stubborn. There is a bullheaded quality to their interpretation of events. There is a single-mindedness in their approach to life. First, they view life through the lens of self. Then they conclude that whatever they think is correct. Finally, they cling to that self-centered opinion no matter what. Safety is often maintained through being stubborn, which is a fiercely loyal protection of self. New suggestions are met with disbelief. "If I didn't think of it, it isn't important to me!" New ideas are dismissed with a degree of scoffing. "That's dumb! That's the dumbest thing I ever heard!" Socially disabled persons are skeptical. "That won't work." End of discussion. Socially disabled individuals dig in their heels and refuse to budge. This underlying stubbornness generates all kind of friction and conflict. A socially disabled parent sees no value in the opinions of children or spouse, and any effort to bring up new ideas is met with sarcasm and hostility. The stubborn socially disabled dyslexic person maintains control through verbal browbeating, nagging, and threatening. There is a stubborn refusal to listen to anything new or different. If a new idea is brought into the relationship, it is pounded into the ground by verbal attack and belittling comments until the other person backs off.

This stubborn characteristic is especially detrimental in our culture today where change is so prevalent and frequent. Since the late 1970s it has been realized that most workers will change jobs or occupations several times before retirement. More than half of all families in the United States will move their place of residence several times. In most occupations new technology makes old job knowledge obsolete within 5 years unless the worker continually learns and grows. Stubborn socially disabled dyslexics do not adapt to such changes. They stubbornly cling to whatever point of view they brought into adult life, and they fight to keep it that way. Socially disabled persons tend to move from job to job, never understanding why boss after boss fires them or lays them off. These stubborn adults think they are being strong by defending a principle. They cannot see the role they play in making it impossible for them to get along. Everyone else is at fault, not them. The job is "dumb" or "the boss is a jerk" or "I just don't want to waste my talent that way." Stubbornness locks the door against letting anything new inside. Stubbornness freezes marriage into a one-sided relationship that gradually squeezes the life out of the spouse. Stubbornness builds a wall between parent and child so that no communication can occur. Eventually the child stops trying to reach the stubborn parent at all. Stubbornness drives wedges between coworkers and colleagues, creating division that eventually causes a work group to fall apart. The stubborn person is soon left behind as society moves forward and new technology makes old ways obsolete. But the stubborn, socially disabled dyslexic does not see it realistically. He or she is right, and everyone else is wrong.

Stubbornness begins as a defense gesture in the dyslexic child. Being stubborn is based upon fear, as we saw in Chapter 5. Youngsters freeze when they are too afraid or unsure to step ahead. An overly fearful child continually freezes. If adults push a fearful child, the youngster balks and sometimes lashes back. This is defensive behavior which thoughtful adults study and usually understand. Why is this bright child refusing to cooperate? Is the child afraid? If so, what is causing the fear? Thoughtful parents and teachers find ways to help the stubborn child release the fear so that forward progress can occur. Dyslexic children are afraid of many things, as Chapter 5 described. Virtually everything the dyslexic child attempts poses a high risk of failure. Those who work with learning disabled children recognize how often dyslexics freeze and feel immobilized. This is defensive behavior that protects the child from too much failure. It is better to be scolded for not trying than to face the scolding that comes from failure. The habits of being stubborn are established early.

Unfortunately, not all parents and teachers know how to deal successfully with childhood stubbornness. Certain adults continue to push too hard. They say: "No child is going to get the best of me!" So the contest of wills is on. W. Hugh Missildine, a psychiatrist, has developed the concept of the "Over-coerced Syndrome" (Missildine & Galton, 1972). He describes this pattern as the ultimately stubborn child who digs in the heels and refuses to budge when adults press for obedience. The more adults press, the more the child refuses. Extremely stubborn children are seen as those who have been pushed too hard too many times while they were afraid. Later they have the automatic habit of digging in the heels in stubborn resistance when any kind of adult pressure is felt or anticipated. The socially disabled dyslexic usually fits this pattern of extreme stubbornness even when there is no reason to display such an attitude. Things simply must go this person's way, or there will be no cooperation. It is a highly successful form of control. Those who must live with this socially disabled individual either give in and do things that way, or they can leave. The stubborn one does not change or yield.

Since stubbornness originates in childhood fear, it is possible to guide fearful children not to be stubborn. The process must begin early, as we have seen before. Adults must recognize the signs of fear in the balking child. What do we do when someone is overly afraid? Intelligent reaction to fear is a quiet, thoughtful discussion of that fear. "What exactly is causing you to be afraid, John?" "I don't know." "Are you afraid because it's dark?" "No." "Are you afraid because Daddy is not home yet?" "Yes," John blurts out. Or he may only nod his head. "OK. I'm glad to know how you feel. Come here and sit in my lap. Let's talk about it. Did you know that Daddy called while you were outside playing? Did you know that he asked how John is this afternoon? Did you know that when the big hand gets to six and the little hand is at nine, Daddy will be home?" As John quietly hears all of these facts, he relaxes and is no longer afraid. Now he is ready to eat supper and be ready to give Daddy a big hug at 9:30. This is the way thoughtful parents walk fearful children through the many moments of fear that spring up during childhood. Teachers work in similar ways to disarm fearful dyslexics at school. John freezes when the class is asked to write the alphabet. He stares out the window and will not lift his pencil. The teacher quietly watches for a while, then she comes over to his desk and bends down. "You know, John," she says quietly. "I wonder something. Has your pencil forgotten how to write *A?*" John nods. "Well, that's no problem. Here, let me help you teach your pencil how to write *A*. Pick up your pencil. That's right. Now I'm going to hold your hand around your pencil. Now let's teach your pencil to write *A*. Oh, yes, that's very good. Now see if your pencil remembers how to write *B*." And John is at work without being afraid of failing.

It takes great courage for a fearful person to move ahead. "What if I fail? What if I don't know how? What if I look dumb? What if someone laughs at me or criticizes me?" All of these questions must be put to rest before fear relaxes and allows forward progress. The stubbornness of social disability is born from this kind of self-questioning. It is possible to teach children how to turn such questions into forward steps if the process begins early enough and continues over a period of time. Stubbornness must be faced in so many areas: how one dresses for school; doing chores instead of playing at that moment; tasting new food; meeting new people; giving up worn-out clothes and toys; letting Mom rearrange the furniture in the room; sharing things with others; letting brother or sister use your stuff; submitting to authority; following a bunch of rules; bowing your head when someone prays; combing your hair when you're 8 years old; taking a shower every night when you're 9 years old; doing homework when you have forgotten how; handing in extra papers when you don't like the teacher. Wise parents and teachers guide youngsters through these developmental steps, a "baby step" at a time. Over a period of years, stubbornness is replaced by courage and willingness to try because fear has been removed through understanding. Nagging, yelling, and criticizing do not remove the stain of stubbornness. These adult responses only grind in the stain more deeply. The stubborn child must be shown how not to be afraid, then he or she must be shown how to move ahead successfully. This cannot be achieved by shouting orders from the sidelines or roughly shoving the fearful child from the back.

Arrogance

Perhaps the most offensive characteristic of social disability is arrogance. The socially disabled person is self-centered, as we have seen. This person is also stubborn and feels a lot of self-pity. He or she can also be arrogant. This is often the last straw in causing relationships to break apart. Self-centered persons are often charming. Self-pitying persons often attract sympathy by appearing cuddly and needing lots of hugs. But the arrogant person is abrasive and cold in his or her display of superiority. The arrogant pattern proclaims: "I am the best. I am the smartest. If you want to know, just ask me. Anyone who disagrees with me is dumb and stupid." An arrogant attitude places others in the embarrassing position of not being bright or competent. The arrogant socially disabled person brags and struts with no regard for the feelings of others. Any conversation is controlled and dominated by a nonstop monologue about self: "I did this; I saw that; I said such and such." The opinions of others are dismissed with a condescending tone because they do not matter. No one else is as wise as this person. No one else has the right answer. This arrogant person is a social bully who intimidates others to get his or her own way. The socially disabled person with an arrogant attitude quickly becomes labeled as a "know-it-all" and is laughed about behind his or her back. Yet the person is blind to this social reaction of others. The socially arrogant person truly believes himself or herself to be superior.

Such a person is a social misfit, unable to fit successfully into groups. This person cannot find acceptance in the usual social ways. This outsider soon tries to develop his or her own group where he or she is in control. It is interesting to watch the arrogant, socially disabled dyslexic person work out strategies for gaining a network of followers. Relationships are based upon the pretense that this person is special and that he or she has something unique the others do not have. We frequently see highly charismatic persons manage successfully for years in this kind of arrogant role. Within the group, there may be intense loyalty that defends the arrogant leader and explains away all of his or her rudeness. This type of leader views others with contempt, but at the same time others are stroked and groomed in ways to make them feel important. The arrogant person uses others, taking whatever they can give without giving in return. This type of person seeks out others who are weak and vulnerable and need to be associated with someone who represents power. These power groups are seen at every level: the playground at school, street corners in large cities, corporate boardrooms, religious organizations, the world of politics. Arrogance uses others, devalues the worth of others, degrades the dignity of others, and stifles the growth of others. Arrogant, socially disabled persons are among the least loved of all members of society, yet they never understand why. They are blind when it comes to seeing how their behavior offends so many others.

Among the elements of social disability, arrogance is one of the most difficult to change. Occasionally we see an arrogant child who is rude, thoughtless, and insensitive. There was much arrogance in Joe, the boy described at the beginning of this chapter. He truly thought that he deserved special treatment because he was very bright. He used his friendship with me to brag to friends about being "Dr. Jordan's special friend." He could not keep from making cutting remarks whenever he observed a mistake or weakness in others. He could not keep his tongue from saying "I told you so" in an arrogant way that instantly aroused others to anger. The car he drove was better than that of anyone else. His coat cost more than anyone else's coat. His gold chain was more valuable. His dad made more money. His brother was the smartest at the university. Girls liked him better than they did other guys, even though he could not keep a relationship going very long. Someday he was going to have his doctorate and make a lot of money. Joe never could see how this arrogant litany provoked others and made him the target of ridicule. He had no friends. No one his own age would associate with him, and he never knew why. It was impossible for him to accept any level of constructive criticism, because he flew into a defensive rage: "There you go, criticizing me like my folks always do!" When the root of arrogance is not changed during a child's formative years, it becomes an obnoxious weed that makes the socially disabled person offensive and unable to fit into normal society. The depth of loneliness is incredible when the arrogant, socially disabled person stops pretending and actually looks for companionship. Persons like Joe suffer deeply when they let down their guard, but they cannot understand why.

How does an arrogant person learn to be humble? In most instances it seems impossible, once the root of arrogance becomes deeply embedded. To be arrogant is to be blind to others, seeing only self. How does one see others when one cannot see? Perhaps the ultimate definition of humility was penned by C.S. Lewis as he developed the concepts of *The Screwtape Letters:* "The truly humble man never thinks of himself at all." I have never known a person who fully met that standard. However, it is possible to help a child with an arrogant attitude begin to change, if the teaching process begins soon enough. This transformation from being egocentric to recognizing the worth of others starts with "baby steps" that show the child how to look at others realistically. Instead of blurting out the judgment that "Jack is dumb! He's really stupid!" Joe is guided through a discussion. "No, Joe. Jack isn't dumb. He is just as intelligent as you. Have you ever noticed that certain things are hard for Jack to do? Have you ever noticed how hard he struggles to write well? Watch how hard he must work to write as well as you do." "OK, but I'm better than he is at writing." "That's right, Joe, you are. But Jack is better than you at math. Have you ever noticed that every person is best at something, but nobody is best at everything?" "Well, OK, but it's still dumb the way Jack writes." "No, Joe, we aren't going to call anyone dumb. Do you want people to say you're 'dumb' because you can't remember your multiplication facts?" "No, but that's different!" "No, Joe, it is not different. Writing is easier for you than it is for Jack, but math is easier for him than it is for you. We aren't going to call each other dumb, Joe. That just is not acceptable."

This kind of patient teaching bears good results over a period of time if the arrogant child receives this model from at least two sources. Yet if he sees it from only one source, while he sees an arrogant, sarcastic, overly critical pattern in other sources, he does not change his tendencies and the root for arrogance continues to grow. The young man Joe whom I have described did not have this kind of patient guidance during his formative years. He followed the models he saw at home and at the private school he attended. His close, supportive relationship with me was not enough to change his bent toward being arrogant. Had either his home or school presented him with the right kind of teaching model and example, then he and I could have worked through his arrogant spirit and he could have learned how to view others in a compassionate way.

Immaturity

Most socially disabled dyslexics are immature. Physically they may reach adult maturity ahead of schedule, but emotionally they remain immature. They tend to be impatient, snapping into anger at the least irritation. They tend to be impulsive, darting off on rabbit trails without thinking about the consequences. They often are not afraid of physical danger, which leaves them without the normal warning signals most of us hear when we are approaching danger. They behave much less maturely than most people their age, causing them to be misfits with peers. They usually have short attention span so that they become bored too soon to enjoy typical activities. They tend to be shallow spiritually, having no interest in developing deeper understanding of faith or religious teaching. They are often materialistic in that they want all kinds of nice things but do not have the income to afford that life-style. They tend to be jealous, which makes them impossible partners in romantic relationships or friendships. They often are insatiable, never achieving full satisfaction no matter how much attention or affection they receive. They tend to wear out their relationships too quickly by being overly demanding and possessive. They are insecure, fretting over little issues that most people realize are minor. They tend to clamor, fret, fuss, beg, demand, accuse, blow up, have tantrums, waste what they have, and live dangerously. Socially disabled persons often "act like babies" in situations in which their peers remain calm and mature.

In evaluating the learning patterns of dyslexic students, we usually find wide differences between their highest areas of ability and their lowest areas of performance. For example, most dyslexics are quite intelligent. Mental age is usually higher than chronological age. Reading age (grade level at which students can read successfully) is usually well below mental age. Work stamina age (a measure of ability to stay with school work without becoming restless and disruptive) is usually far below mental age. Emotional maturity age (level of self-control and ability to put off satisfying a wish) is also far below the level of intelligence. For instance, a dyslexic boy who is also socially disabled might have the following profile:

Mental age	12
Chronological age	10½
Reading age	8
Work stamina age	7
Emotional maturity age	6½

This means that in a quiet, one-to-one situation with a tutor or instructor, this boy displays the brightness and intelligence we would expect of most 12-year-olds, although his age is only 10½. However, in the classroom, he handles reading assignments with the skills we see in most beginning third graders. At age 10½ he is in fifth grade, which means that he cannot handle silent reading tasks at that level. His reading skills are more than 2 years below expected ability level.

As teachers try to work with his group, this child begins to fidget, squirm, and interrupt as a young 7-year-old child would do in early second grade. Compared with his fifth-grade classmates, this boy is immature and disruptive, always off on rabbit trails instead of keeping his attention focused on the task. When it comes to emotional control, he reacts to stress as if he were 6½ years old. He flares too easily, whines too much, complains too often, begs, and wheedles. He bursts into tears at a certain point of frustration. He is like an overwhelmed 6½-year-old child trying to cope with fifth-grade classroom work.

Older persons who are socially disabled have the same kind of wide disparity between their highest abilities and their level of emotional control. Being immature means that they cannot cope with life at the level of their age. Young adults who are socially disabled will not carry out responsibility. They cannot be depended upon to keep promises, show up for work on time, help out when they agreed, pay their share of expenses, pay bills on time, save money instead of spending, or deny themselves immediate pleasure so that something better can be enjoyed later. They give in to whatever whim or impulse bubbles up at the moment. If they have $50.00 to pay on the rent, they may spend it all for beer or a good time on Saturday, then be in trouble for not having rent money on Monday. If they promise to meet someone at a certain time, they may not show up or bother to call. Something else more immediate came up and they forgot their appointment. If they have a job interview at 9:00, they may oversleep and not wake up until noon, then they do not understand when someone else gets the job. On the job they look for the easy way out and try to avoid doing whatever the boss assigned. If these immature misfits get married, they are like disorganized children playing house. If a child is born to the marriage, the socially disabled parent is no more able to cope with the demands of parenthood than a 12-year-old would be. Most of the cases of child abuse occur when socially disabled adults try to rear children. The crying of the child, the normal mess of changing diapers, the need to earn a steady income to provide food and medical care for the baby, all such responsibilities are too much for the immature, socially disabled adult. Without warning this person bursts into a tantrum and tries to make the baby stop crying or stop being a nuisance. A great deal of physical abuse toward the spouse or mate occurs with these immature adults. All their lives they have thrown tantrums. They have slammed doors and squealed tires and gunned their car at a hundred miles an hour when they were angry. They carry these tantrum habits into marriage, onto the job, or into any relationship they try to have. The immature, socially disabled person cannot cope with adult life except on a childish level.

How do parents and teachers tame this kind of explosive immaturity? Is it possible to turn this strongly emotional life response a different way? If the process begins early enough, as we have seen in this chapter, immaturity can be modified enough to give the person at least the basic social skills of self-control. When an impulsive, immature child throws a tantrum, adults face certain choices. The adult can fly at the child and spank, slap, or otherwise punish the child physically. This often stops the tantrum, but it also is force meeting force. The adult has stooped to the child's emotional level. The adult tantrum has won over that of the child. Peace may have been restored, but the child has the model of hitting when one is angry. Only now the child dares not hit the "larger child" because the angry adult will hit back. Occasionally it is appropriate for an adult to shock an angry child into breaking the tantrum. Sometimes a swat on the rear is the best thing to do at the moment. But the habit of hitting the child who is having a tantrum is not the model we wish to present when we think of teaching the child how to become mature later on.

When children behave immaturely, they must see mature behavior acted out. They must have clear models of what it means to have patience, to forgive, to maintain self-control, and not to hit back. This requires enormous patience over a long period of time. This does not mean that the adult is not firm or decisive. Dealing with an immature, angry, or impulsive child requires a great deal of firm, decisive adult control. The point is that the adult stays in charge in a way that leads the child through the moment of immaturity, then a discussion follows. "John, why were you so angry?" "He got my toy." "But you have a lot of toys. Just look at all of the toys you have to play with." "I want that toy. He can't have it!" "No, John, that is not how we do with our toys. We have to share. Did Jim jerk your toy away from you?" "No, but I wanted it next." "You mean that you were not playing with it when Jim took it?" "No, but it's mine! I want it! He can't have it!" "No, John. It is Jim's turn to play with the toy. You have another toy to play with. Later on Jim will let you play with his toy." If this type of patient rehearsal does not work, then John is firmly taken someplace else. He may be taken to his room if he is at home, or to a different part of the classroom if he is at school. His tantrum does not cause the adult to let him have his way. Over and over during his developmental years, John receives this type of firm, reasonable guidance. The adult gives him something else to do, whenever possible, but the child's temper does not prevail. His tantrum does not make Jim give up the toy because John demands it.

As immature children grow up, thoughtful parents and teachers require certain amounts of responsibility. Parents make written lists of chores, then they guide the child in doing everything on the lists.

Teachers write lists of assignments, then they guide the child in doing every task on the lists. As parents and teachers work together, the immature child begins to understand that a certain amount of structure must be followed. The child may not like structure, but he or she learns that it has to be done. Sometimes a reward is the right way to motivate a child to finish responsibilities. Sometimes taking away a privilege is the only discipline he or she will understand. Parents or teachers may have to ground the immature child if certain rules are ignored or disobeyed. Over a period of time, this type of structure instills a sense of responsibility within the child's emerging set of values. Like it or not, certain things simply must be done before personal wishes will be fulfilled.

Dyslogic Behavior

In the early 1970s John Wacker intrigued the clinical world when he published a monograph entitled *The Dyslogic Syndrome* (Wacker, 1975). After many years of struggling with his daughter's learning problems, he outlined for the first time a pattern of irregular behaviors we see in many socially disabled adults. Earlier in this chapter we read a summary of research about right-brain lesions and how they produce a type of illogical, "weird" behavior in a certain number of our struggling young people (Right Hemi Syndrome). Wacker pioneered the concept of the Dyslogic Syndrome, which now is seen as a brain-based problem that partially blocks a person's ability to live by common sense reasoning or logical thinking.

Dyslogic behavior is very upsetting to anyone involved in that person's life. As the word implies, the person does not do things in a normal, logical way. Decisions are often totally unpredictable and irrational. This person may suddenly sell his car for $300.00 after working 18 months and making $1,500.00 in payments. A dyslogic girl may drop out of school within a semester of graduation to work part-time for minimum wage. Her explanation is that she got bored with school and wanted to start her career. It makes no sense that she is now earning $65.00 a week at a burger place. A dyslogic boy may suddenly quit his job 2 days after being promoted to assistant manager. "I just got tired of it," he explains. "How are you going to keep up your car payments and your insurance?" his father asks. "Oh, it will work out," he says as he dashes off to have a party with his buddies. We often see two dyslogic young people marry, which sets into motion a marriage without any kind of structure or logical foundation. They begin to run up debts on charge accounts. They buy expensive items on impulse. They party all night and sleep all day. They do not clean house or do dishes. They fight all the time, yet they are extremely jealous if one spouse flirts with another person. It is impossible for parents to reason with the dyslogic youngster. They do not think in a logical way. They do not respond to logical thinking. They have no regard for tradition that expects everyone in society to be responsible. They have no intention of "dancing the tribal dance," yet they demand to have all the comforts modern society offers. They demand that parents give them money or pay their bills or bail them out of trouble. Yet they refuse to work things out through counseling. These dyslogical socially disabled young people are too loose to establish productive lives. They do not follow guidance. They cannot live by a schedule. They cannot follow through on responsibility. They get themselves into astonishing problem situations with no plans for getting out. They live entirely by the impulse of the moment. And they are beyond our reach when it comes to logical appeals or common sense reasoning.

Is it possible to turn dyslogic behavior another way? As further study is done of the brain structures of dyslexics, we realize that the learning disability of dyslexia is a left-brain condition with which many children are born. Many dyslexics gradually outgrow enough of the pattern to become successful later on, although they must always deal with poor spelling, poor math computation, and faulty reading. Some dyslexics are too severely handicapped ever to attain literacy skills, but they can become successful adults with the right kind of guidance during their formative years. Those who also display the Dyslogic Syndrome present an even more difficult problem. If dyslogic behavior is largely caused by lesions within the right-brain hemisphere, then the disruptive, illogical behavior I have described is beyond the reach of counseling or advice. If it is caused largely by neurological dysfunction, then the dyslogic person has little control over the weird, irregular behavior that makes his or her life so unstable.

If dyslogic behavior is recognized early enough, it can be modified somewhat, although the person will always be prone to impulsive decisions and irregular behavior. If firm behavior modification is begun in childhood when the dyslogical child is still teachable and guidable, it is possible to implant enough awareness of cause and effect to enable him or her to succeed by the early adult years. However, it is impossible to erase the dyslogic thinking patterns altogether. The key is to maintain very tight structure over a period of years so the struggling youngster is kept within certain boundaries. Every fence, every restriction, every adult limitation is clearly labeled and the reasons why are made clear. "No, Jason. You may not ride your bike over to Allen's house." "Why not? Jim gets to ride his bike anywhere he wants!" "No, Jason. Your brother does not ride anywhere he wants, and you know that. The reason you may not ride your bike to Allen's house is that you do not pay attention to traffic. Until you learn to stop and look carefully, we are not going to let you ride your bike that far. And that is how it is going to be." No amount of complaining, threatening, or fussing changes the rule. So long as Jason's behavior is illogical or exposes him to danger, then his behavior will be supervised and controlled. As he matures, he is held responsible for paying for things he breaks. He must apologize whenever he is rude. He must face up to the part he plays when things get out of hand or he creates difficulty. He is not allowed to get away with blaming others, demanding his own way, saying hateful things out of spite, acting out jealous feelings, having money to splurge on whims, and so forth.

Baby step by baby step, Jason learns certain lessons as he grows up. He learns that if he is immature, he will be disciplined like a younger child. He learns that if he creates an expensive loss of some kind, he must pay for the damage. He learns that he must earn a certain amount of money before he can make certain purchases. He learns that, whether he likes it or not, there are limits. He learns that there are laws governing society, and there are police officers who enforce those laws. He learns that Mom and Dad do not take his side against teachers, unless a certain teacher was clearly unfair. He learns that a family must maintain a certain level of courtesy and mutual respect. He learns that beyond a certain point, his parents do not give him money or pay the bills he accumulates. He learns that he cannot get away with using people. He learns that he must give a certain amount if he hopes to receive. These basic social lessons can be learned if adults do not wait too late. But the Dyslogic Syndrome described by Wacker is impossible to change completely. Right-brain research is showing increasing evidence that the underlying cause for this irregular behavior lies within the brain structure itself.

Becoming Independent

Being independent means that people can handle life alone without help. They can make personal decisions without a supervisor or advisor. They can plan ahead and work toward goals without being supervised. They can make decisions that are based upon common sense reasoning and therefore carry them toward a more comfortable life with the help of parents. Being independent means that we may turn to friends or parents for their opinion, but we do not have to have the approval of others to know what to do. Being independent means cutting childhood roots to a certain degree and replanting one's life with new concepts that do not depend upon what Mom or Dad say or do. To be independent, one must be able to read all of the signs and do what they say without having to ask an interpreter for help. An independent person still enjoys talking things over with a trusted advisor, because being independent includes knowing the value of wisdom. Being independent means one can make decisions, change plans, establish new values, and start on new journeys without needing the help of anyone else.

It is difficult for dyslexics to reach this level of independence. As we saw in Chapter 5, many dyslexic persons marry someone who becomes the "parent" or "supervisor" to keep life structured as Mom and Dad used to do. Most dyslexic adults feel more comfortable and a great deal safer if there is someone nearby, ready to help when things are not clear. It is not actually necessary for a dyslexic person to become fully independent, as I have described above. One need not be totally alone and independent in order to have a satisfactory life. But a certain degree of independence must be achieved if a dyslexic man or woman is to become a fulfilled adult with positive self-esteem and a good self-image.

Certain basic skills must be mastered if dyslexics are to become independent of parents as they enter the adult world. As we saw in Chapter 5, dyslexics tend to go one of four ways as they emerge into their twenties. Most dyslexics find a partner who can provide enough support and structure to make the transition into adulthood successful. Others are not ready until much later to leave home and establish life for themselves. Some drift out into the world as loners, living alone with little or no contact with society beyond a few narrow areas. Some become involved with illegal activity to the point of becoming wards of the court. This group includes many dyslogic persons who cannot manage the rules of society successfully. However, if one is to become a successfully independent person, one must learn certain skills.

Time Awareness

In earlier chapters we have studied the basic problem dyslexics have with time concepts. Few dyslexics ever develop a clear, sustained mental image of time segments and how they occur in sequence. This means that dyslexic men and women must live by visible time schedules that provide a structure they can follow. Most dyslexics need two forms of time chart, a pocket log that they carry at all times, and a larger calendar on which they jot down appointments and dates they must remember. Over a period of time, these forms of time reminders become refined enough to fit each dyslexic person's individual style. The pocket log must show time in weekly and monthly segments. Pages are arranged so that each week is divided into days, and each day is divided into hours. Space is provided to write appointments for each hour of each day of each week of the month. The dyslexic adult then learns to follow this pocket guide. Most dyslexics develop their own "shorthand" symbols or codes for writing essential information. Often no one else can interpret these notations. But they are the lifeline of dyslexics, keeping them anchored in the stream of events as they move through time. Without this daily log, dyslexic adults forget appointments, overlook events that are important to the family, and so forth. At home or on the job, dyslexics also keep a calendar that shows long-range obligations such as birthdays, future apointments, and deadlines. Earlier chapters have described the importance of training children to use these kinds of time awareness procedures. When dyslexics are prepared to keep track of time, they have taken the first step toward becoming independent. It is a tragic mistake for adults to allow dyslexic young people to drift into their adult years without this kind of careful preparation to manage time. It is sad to see intelligent dyslexic adults struggling on their own with no skills in managing time expectations.

Living Skills

No dyslexic man or woman can become independent until he or she knows how to do basic chores such as simple housekeeping, cooking, laundry, and shopping. It is essential that parents use the developmental years of childhood and adolescence to teach dyslexics to live alone someday. Even if reading ability is too limited to permit them to cook from a recipe, severely dyslexic young people can learn to prepare nutritious meals in a microwave oven. Parents should spend the high school years training dyslexic teenagers to shop for basic food items that can be prepared without needing a recipe. It is highly important that junk food items be avoided and that balanced eating habits be established. Microwave cooking is quick and simple with today's variety of foods available. Potatoes can be baked in a few minutes. Fresh vegetables can be steamed if the person is taught a few basic procedures. Even eggs can be prepared in a microwave oven with certain utensils. There is no excuse for a teen becoming an adult knowing only how to pop corn or warm up a TV dinner in the microwave oven. Being an independent adult means that the dyslexic knows how to prepare simple nutritious meals even when reading skills are limited.

It is equally essential for dyslexics to know how to keep house well enough to avoid living in squalor. All young people should be taught to make beds, do laundry, clean up the apartment once a week, do dishes or use the dishwasher, clean the bathroom occasionally, and so forth. Dyslexic men must be able to invite friends over without being ashamed of their place. This includes learning the mysteries of doing one's own laundry and not taking it home for Mom to do every weekend. There is an important sense of pride in helping dyslexics become independent in their personal affairs without needing to depend on Mom or someone else for basic needs. Keeping house adequately is as important as earning a living or finishing an eduation. The self-esteem of dyslexics is greatly enhanced when they can keep their own place without needing help.

Managing Money

Probably the most difficult task for dyslexics to learn is how to manage money. Those with poor arithmetic skills often struggle with the addition and subtraction involved in writing checks and keeping a checking account untangled. At times dyslexics need help with that kind of bookkeeping. But it is essential that they learn how to handle money for themselves. This process must begin by early teens. Wise parents open a checking account for the dyslexic child at about age 14. The child is paid a certain "salary" each month that includes school lunch fees, special fees for classes, a certain amount for clothing, and any other fixed expenses during the month. A simple budget is written so that the child sees what must be spent, when it will be spent, and how much money will be left after all bills are paid. The ideal system shows the child how to write checks for school lunches, clothing purchases, and any other purchase where a check is appropriate. Mom or Dad supervises this procedure, helping the child learn to write a check successfully. The child is not expected to balance the checkbook alone, but when the statement arrives each month, he or she watches while the adult does so. If the child takes a part-time job, those earnings are deposited in the checking account, as well as in a savings account if that is appropriate. The point is to guide children step by step as they handle their own money. Over a period of 5 or 6 years, the dyslexic learns how to be independent in handling money. Mom and Dad no longer have to do all of the work or make all of the decisions. If the dyslexic child is immature and impulsive, this self-control system helps greatly by teaching what happens when the account is overdrawn or when lunch money is spent for something else. The child is responsible, not the adult. This kind of planning prepares the dyslexic to step out into the adult world ready to be independent with money management. The absence of this kind of training guarantees that the dyslexic person will be crippled when it is time to face the demands of adult life.

Holding a Job

It is almost too late if a dyslexic young person does not work until after high school. Holding a job involves far more than earning money or putting in a certain number of hours during the week. Holding a job requires a certain level of social skill, the ability to get along with coworkers, the ability to follow instructions, and the ability to please a boss. Many dyslexics must learn these skills over a period of time. These basic survival lessons must begin during the early teen years or before. If a dyslexic child is immature, socially disabled, or dyslogical, it will be very difficult for him or her to master job skills. Youngsters who are obviously immature may not be employable if they cannot fit into a job situation successfully. However, as soon as the child is capable of carrying out job responsibility, he or she should begin part-time work. This usually requires a great deal of patient help from parents. Occasionally dyslexic youngsters are self-assured enough to find jobs on their own. Usually parents need to walk them through the steps of locating possible jobs, interviewing the employer, filling out necessary forms, and having dependable transportation. Then parents must be willing to stay in touch with these new workers, talking things over to make sure they are handling the job expectations well enough and helping them interpret on-the-job situations accurately. Occasionally parents must step in as advocates if they realize that dyslexia has caused the child to misperceive something important at work. It is essential to give dyslexic teens this kind of sheltered experience rather than assuming that they should wait until they are older to begin the work process. The sooner they enter the world of working and earning wages, the better prepared they will be to become independent as they finish school.

Dealing with Problems

Few parents or teachers realize that dyslexics need a great deal of coaching over a period of time in how to handle conflict effectively.

More mature dyslexics work out their own ways of resolving conflict without needing outside help. Many do not. Again, fear is a major factor as a dyslexic person under pressure faces an adversary or is forced to continue in a situation where he or she would rather not continue. Most dyslexics will meet someone on the job who makes life miserable. The easy way out is to quit, but this often leads to the habit of quitting at the first sign of conflict. Dyslexics who feel a lot of fear must learn how to handle those feelings without running away or giving up. Parents do not always know from surface behavior what is bothering the youngster. What appears to be anger may actually be fear that is eating the student alive. What appears to be "leave me alone" behavior may actually be gnawing fear that the student does not know how to express. He or she may be overwhelmed by humiliation and unable to express it in words. The child may feel too intimidated or threatened by a bully to say anything at all. Parents must be alert for signs of drawing back or wanting to quit. Adults must be patient instead of critical until the issues are out in the open. It is of great importance that dyslexic teens learn to work through these issues while they are still at home. Waiting until their adult years to learn these lessons of the marketplace may be too late. It is impossible to become independent if one cannot handle conflict or deal with problems without help.

7

Adults Who Have Overcome Dyslexia

As we have seen in earlier chapters, not all dyslexics overcome their problems to become successful. Many are too scarred by childhood experiences to have the courage or inner strength to overcome their disabilities. For many, life circumstances overwhelm their ambitions, crushing their hopes and dreams. Yet many dyslexics do break through the barriers that block their way. As they pass through their teens and enter their early adult years, they find ways to compensate, bypass permanent learning disabilities, and achieve victories that may have seemed impossible in early years. How does a dyslexic person overcome such a deep-seated, life-saturating condition? How do certain individuals emerge from years of struggle and near failure as happy, creative adults? Why do some dyslexics succeed when classmates and peers with the same kind of handicap do not? This is an intriguing story that has been told by many successful adults as they reflect on the hurdles they have crossed. It is greatly encouraging to ponder the stories of dyslexics who have succeeded. There are valuable lessons in courage and hope as they tell their victory stories. In Chapter 5 we heard from Jay, the unstable dyslexic boy who had no stories to tell. Now we shall hear some exciting victory stories from adults who overcame their language disabilities in remarkable ways.

An interesting controversy exists among professionals as to whether it is permissible to discuss learning disability, dyslexia, or dysfunctional language patterns in historical figures no longer living. For example, the *Journal of Learning Disabilities* reflects the wide differences of opinion surrounding this idea. Volume 4, Number 1 (January 1971, pp. 34–45) presents a fascinating article by Lloyd J. Thompson, MD, from Chapel Hill, North Carolina, entitled "Language Disabilities in Men of Eminence." Dr. Thompson discussed his findings as he researched handwritten documents, diaries, publications, and personal interviews of relatives of such historical persons as Thomas Edison, Harvey Cushing, Woodrow Wilson, Auguste Rodin, and Albert Einstein. Dr. Thompson's article includes his theories regarding what causes dyslexia, to which he attributed the language disabilities of most of his men of eminence. Volume 20, Number 5 (May 1982, pp. 270–279) of the *Journal of Learning Disabilities* presented an article by Kimberly A. Adelman and Howard S. Adelman. These writers refute Dr. Thompson's earlier opinions on the basis that he did not have clear-cut clinical evidence of dyslexia in his subjects. My point is that equally intelligent points of view exist on both sides of this issue. Regardless of whether we apply posthumous labels such as *dyslexia* or *language disability,* we can see clear evidence of struggle with language skills in the lives of such persons. It is helpful to see how such persons of history overcame their language processing handicaps enough to achieve success.

Thomas Alva Edison

Like many dyslexics through the years, Thomas A. Edison barely survived the first years of childhood. Nancy Edison was 37 years old when this son was born. She had already lost three children through miscarriage, and she was determined that this last child should survive. Thomas was somewhat deformed at birth with an overly large head. His early motor and language skills were very slow to emerge. Physicians of that day advised his parents that the child had suffered from "brain fever" and would always be an "invalid." It is recorded that relatives, friends, neighbors, and professionals of that day advised Nancy Edison to "put him away" and not to hope that he would ever be normal. When Thomas was sent to school, he was diagnosed as "mentally ill" because he could not do the academic work expected at that time. Mrs. Edison became enraged over that diagnosis. She withdrew her struggling son from school and vowed to teach him at home by herself. When Thomas was 7 years old, he contracted scarlet fever, which set into motion the gradual deafness that cost him his hearing by his early adult years.

During Edison's childhood, adults labeled him as "backward" and "addled." He strongly resented such labels, and he turned to his mother as his main source for knowledge. As Mrs. Edison, who was a former teacher, developed ways to help her son learn, Mr. Edison became strongly disappointed in his "retarded son" and refused to pay for extra things, leaving mother and son on their own to work out an educational program the best they could. From time to time Thomas returned to public school, but he was never able to fit into a classroom structure. In his later years he wrote: "I remember I used never to be able to get along in school. I was always at the foot of the class.... My father thought that I was stupid, and I almost decided that I was a dunce."

Throughout his developmental years, Thomas listened as his mother read to him. Through listening he absorbed great quantities of literature, history, science, philosophy, the Bible, and whatever else Mrs. Edison could add to his knowledge. This home-school education nurtured the boy's hunger for knowledge, but he did not develop traditional literacy skills. A biography by Josephson *(Edison, A Biography,* McGraw-Hill, 1959) describes Thomas's literacy skills as follows: "Her son never learned how to spell; up to the time of his manhood his grammar and syntax were appalling. We see that he was hard to teach. Whatever he learned, he learned in his own way. In fact, though his mother inspired him, no one ever taught him anything; he taught himself."

At age 19 Thomas Edison wrote a letter to his mother: "Dear Mother. Started the Store several weeks. I have growed considerably I don't look much like a Boy now—How all the folk did you receive a Box of Books from Memphis that he promised to send them—languages. You son Al." Thomas kept a diary most of his adult life. As he grew older, he developed a simple writing style that allowed him to express his thoughts clearly, but he always used simple words, short sentences, and brief wording. He avoided words that he could not spell.

At age 67 Edison wrote an essay that revealed his deep, often bitter feelings toward public education. In 1914 he said:

> I am frequently asked about our system of education. I say that we have none. Our system is a relic of the past. It consists of parrot-like repetitions. It is a dull study of twenty-six hieroglyphs. Groups of hieroglyphs. That is what the young of this present day study. Here is an object. I place it in the hands of a child. I tell him to look at it.... Why should we make him take impressions of things through the ear when he may be able to

> see? . . . It is of the utmost importance that every faculty should meet the environment. What is the use of crowding the mind with facts which cannot be utilized by the child because the method of their acquisition is distasteful to him?
>
> I like the Montessori method. It teaches through play. It makes learning a pleasure. . . . That system of education will succeed which shows to those who learn the actual thing—not the ghost of it. I firmly believe that the motion picture is destined to bear an important part in the education of the future.

The fertile mind of Thomas Alva Edison, which gave the world so many life-changing inventions, realized the value of multisensory learning for children. He had achieved his knowledge by developing multisensory techniques and strategies that allowed him to connect several sensory pathways at the same time. He realized that rote memory was not the best way to teach children, especially those who struggled with silent learning the traditional way.

Edison displayed numerous signs of dyslexia. What was the key to his success? Early in his life, Edison became angry, and his anger became the primary drive that allowed him to conquer his language disabilities. His intelligent mother was able to channel this anger in productive ways so that he did not waste his potential just being angry. He learned to move ahead in spite of being rejected by his father and being hideously labeled by his school. For Edison, anger turned the right way was the key to future success. In his later years, he no longer needed anger to drive him forward, but it was the essential ingredient to keep him moving ahead during his difficult formative years.

George S. Patton IV

This famous general of World War II had a most unusual childhood. His father was a strong, domineering man who reared the family in isolation on a ranch. The Patton children were forbidden to mix with other youngsters, and they did not attend school until their teen years. George Patton III strongly believed in oral learning tradition. He thought that no child should learn to read until after age 12. The Patton children were immersed in oral reading. Adults in the family took turns reading aloud from the classics and the Bible. George S. Patton IV spent his first 12 years in this isolated environment, absorbing oral literature the way he breathed air. He had extraordinary memory for what he heard. After hearing an adult read or deliver a speech, he could recite it almost word by word without ever having seen the printed text. He developed a grand style of oratory, strutting about the ranch shouting long poems and passages from literature by the hour. He brought great pride to his father who probably had reading disability himself and therefore had no regard for traditional literacy skills. By his 12th birthday, Patton had the literary education of an adult, all of which was learned orally.

At age 12, Patton was sent to a private school which was designed to prepare him to enter West Point Military Academy. At that time he could not read. He was an authority on world literature and he could write in a unique script, but he could not read. Entering the private preparatory school was a deep shock to his self-esteem. Suddenly he was transplanted from a home environment where he was displayed as a "genius" to a school environment where he was regarded as ignorant. He began to "cheat" by getting information from classmates. He quickly placed himself in the good favor of his instructors by keeping every rule better than anyone else. In the prep school and later at West Point, Patton astonished everyone by his remarkable auditory memory. He could hear a lecture or sermon once, then repeat it verbatim days later. This astounding ability to absorb oral information and retain it over a period of time amazed his peers and leaders.

Patton never became a fluent reader. He compensated through his skills at retaining what he heard. He developed rather irritating "show-off" habits of overwhelming his critics by his phenomenal memory, but he could not read well. He was an avid reader of the Bible, military history, poetry, and certain areas of literature, but his reading was always slow and labored. When he commanded armies during World War II, he was often seen alone, slowly working through the Bible or some other reading material. He muttered it aloud to himself as he slowly sounded out the words and toiled through line after line of print.

How did this brilliant, apparently dyslexic man succeed? Critics of George Patton have been harsh in describing his arrogance and often haughty behavior. His enemies delighted in reminding the world of his famous outbursts of temper, as when he slapped the young soldier across the face for refusing to join the front lines in combat. But those who regarded Patton as a friend recognized an extraordinary drive to succeed. He was a proud man who held certain principles strongly. He had an abiding religious faith which he was not ashamed to proclaim. He never resolved certain hostile feelings toward military leaders who made his life difficult. He needed to prove that he was as good or better than anyone else. He had a driving need to show the world that even if he could not read, he was just as intelligent and just as worthy as any other person. Pride, ambition, and a brilliant capacity to absorb what he heard gave Patton the ability to overcome his language processing difficulties that embarrassed him so deeply during his teen years.

Woodrow Wilson

It seems incredible that a person with language disabilities could become president of a prestigious university, then president of the United States. Yet that is the history of Woodrow Wilson. As the United States entered the 20th century, Woodrow Wilson was president of Princeton University. Soon he was elected president of the United States, in time to guide the country through World War I. Wilson was a young child during the Civil War. Like so many others with dyslexic-like patterns, he was taught at home during his early school years. There he listened to many hours of oral reading from the Bible and classical literature. Woodrow did not learn the alphabet until age 9, and he did not learn to read until age 11. He never did well in school. Those who have researched his life report that he was always a "mediocre student." He tried to avoid subjects that required abstract reading. He soon excelled as a public speaker and won recognition in student debate. By his early adult years he was well known as an orator.

Tommy, as Wilson was called by his family, was ill much of his life. He did not finish high school because of illness, and his college studies were often interrupted by illness. Later he would become fatally ill toward the end of his term in office as president of the United States. Along with having language processing problems, he had to deal with illness that often forced him to drop out of school or change his plans. A major influence during childhood had been his father, who was a minister. The Reverend Wilson spent long hours reading scripture to his son, discussing doctrine, and helping him develop a deep sense of right and wrong. As an adult, Woodrow Wilson carried this spiritual attitude into his career. He exhausted himself working for world peace. He was a major force behind the creation of the League of Nations following World War I. In fact, he no doubt shortened his life as he pressed for his ideals of peace and world brotherhood. Wilson always needed help to express his ideas in writing, but his outstanding speaking skills masked the underlying struggle he always had with reading and spelling.

What was the secret of this language disabled man's success? There is no evidence that Wilson was angry or that he sought to vindicate himself before his critics. His motivation came from deeply held spiritual values. He overcame his language handicaps and poor health in order to make the world a better, more peaceful place for future generations.

Albert Einstein

Of all the famous persons within the last century, perhaps the most surprising to be considered language disabled was Albert Einstein. His son, Albert Einstein, Jr., gave a thoughtful summary of his famous father's early years: "He was even considered backward by his teachers. He told me that his teachers reported to his father that he was mentally slow, unsociable, and adrift forever in his foolish dreams." During his early years, Einstein had very poor speech, which developed far behind usual schedule. His parents feared that this late-developing child was "dull." At one point the boy was dismissed from school and labeled a "dunce" by his exasperated teachers. His speech was always rather slow and labored, which caused him to appear shy. In his later years as a faculty member at Princeton University, Einstein spoke softly and was difficult to understand. In fact, he lost three teaching positions in his late twenties because he could not communicate adequately during lectures.

At age 12 Einstein was barely able to read, and his speech was awkward and difficult to understand. Yet his brilliance began to emerge in mathematics and physics. He often could not verbalize his astonishing concepts of math. His writing at that time was filled with dyslexic-like patterns we now recognize as dysgraphia and poor spelling. His language skills were always poor, even while his skills in higher math soared beyond the understanding of all but a few of the world's scholars. Einstein remained a private, very shy man all his life. Occasionally he blossomed in a public way. He appeared in commercial advertisements during his tenure as professor at Princeton University, and his unique personal appearance became known worldwide. However, he was never able to verbalize or communicate orally above a limited level.

How could such a shy, sensitive, language disabled man succeed? Albert Einstein had to absorb enormous insult during the first third of his life. This gentle, compassionate man had no way to hold his own in a competitive world in which success is usually measured by how well one can defend his or her territory. This meek, soft-spoken man saw within himself the ability to contribute new knowledge to the world, knowledge that could revolutionize civilization. We will never know the personal pain he endured before his intelligence was finally recognized. Einstein succeeded in spite of language disabilities because he had a new dream. Within himself he had no choice but to follow that dream until it was recognized by the critical world in which he lived. There was no anger or driving ambition behind this man's success. There was enormous strength that gave him the ability to absorb insult, yet keep on trying until he finally caught the attention of others.

Nelson A. Rockefeller

One of the most powerful political figures of the middle 1900s was severely dyslexic. Nelson Rockefeller was four times governor of New York, then was appointed vice president of the United States. In private life he was a philanthropist who gave millions of dollars to improve life for people around the world. His reading disability was so severe he could not read speeches on television. He employed full-time assistants to be with him at all times to help him cope with language situations made difficult by his dyslexia. In 1976 Nelson Rockefeller published a brief biography to promote a nationally televised program about dyslexia. His own words are the best way to understand how this courageous man finally won success:

> Those watching the Public Broadcasting Service program on "The Puzzle Children" (October 19, 1976) will include a very interested Vice President of the United States. For I was one of the "puzzle children" myself—a dyslexic, or "reverse reader"—and I still have a hard time reading today. But after coping with this problem for more than 60 years, I have a message of encouragement for children with learning disabilities and their parents. Based upon my own experience, my message to dyslexic children is this:
>
> —Don't accept anyone's verdict that you are lazy, stupid, or retarded. You may very well be smarter than most other children your age.
>
> —Just remember that Woodrow Wilson, Albert Einstein, and Leonardo da Vinci also had tough problems with their reading.
>
> —You can learn to cope with your problem and turn your so-called disability into a positive advantage. Dyslexia forced me to develop powers of concentration that have been invaluable throughout my career in business, philanthropy and public life. And I've done an enormous amount of public speaking, especially in political campaigns for Governor of New York and President of the United States.
>
> No one ever heard of dyslexia when I discovered as a boy, along about the third grade, that reading was such a difficult chore that I

was in the bottom one-third of my class. None of the educational, medical and psychological help available today for dyslexics was available in those days. We had no special teachers or tutors, no special classes or courses, no special methods of teaching—because nobody understood our problem.

Along with an estimated three million other children, I just struggled to understand words that seemed to garble before my eyes, numbers that came out backwards, and sentences that were hard to grasp.

And so I accepted the verdict of the IQ tests that I wasn't as bright as most of the rest of my class. Fortunately for me, the school (though it never taught me to spell) was an experimental, progressive institution with the flexibility to let you develop your own interests and follow them. I had a wise and understanding counselor (Dr. Otis W. Caldwell). "Don't worry," he said, "just because you're in the lower third of the class. You've got the intelligence. If you just work harder and concentrate more, you can make it." So I learned through self-discipline to concentrate, which in my opinion is essential for a dyslexic. While I could speak French better than the teacher, because I'd learned it as a child, I couldn't conjugate the verbs. I did flunk Spanish—but now I can speak it fluently because I learned it by ear. My best subject was mathematics. I understood the concepts well beyond my grade level. But it took only one reversed number in a column of figures to cause havoc.

When I came close to flunking out in the ninth grade—because I didn't work very hard that year—I decided that I had better follow Dr. Caldwell's advice if I wanted to go to college. I even told my high school girl friend that we would have to stop dating so I could spend the time studying in order to get into Dartmouth College. And I made it by the skin of my teeth. I made it simply by working harder and longer than the rest—eventually learning to concentrate sufficiently to compensate for my dyslexia in reading. I adopted a regimen of getting up at 5 A.M. to study, and studying without fail. And thanks to my concentration and the very competitive nature I was born with, I found my academic performance gradually improving. In my freshman year at Dartmouth, I was even admitted to a third-year physics course. And in the middle of my sophomore year, I received two A's and three B's for the first semester. My father's letters were filled with joy and astonishment.

I owe a great debt to my professors. Most of all, however, I think I owe my academic improvement to my roommate, Johnny French. Johnny and I were exact opposites. He was reticent and had the highest IQ in the class. To me, he was that maddening type who got straight A's with only occasional reference to books or classes. He was absolutely disgusted with my study habits—anybody who got up at five in the morning to hit the books was, well, peculiar. Inevitably, Johnny made Phi Beta Kappa in our Junior year, but my competitive instincts kept me going. We were both elected to senior fellowships and I made Phi Beta Kappa in my senior year. Johnny, of course, had the last word. He announced that he would never wear his PBK key again—that it had lost all meaning.

Looking back over the years, I remember vividly the pain and mortification I felt as a boy of eight when I was assigned to read a short passage of Scripture at a vesper service—and did a thoroughly miserable job of it. I know what a dyslexic child goes through–the frustration of not being able to do what other children do easily, the humiliation of being thought not too bright when such is not the case at all. My personal discoveries as to what is required to cope with dyslexia could be summarized in these admonitions to the individual dyslexic:

—Accept the fact that you have a problem. Don't just try to hide it.

—Refuse to feel sorry for yourself.

—Realize that you don't have an excuse. You have a challenge.

—Face the challenge.

—Work harder and learn mental discipline, the capacity for total concentration.

—Never quit.

If it helps a dyslexic child to know I went through the same thing...

—BUT I can conduct press conferences in three languages

—AND I can read a speech on television—IF I rehearse it six times, with my script in large type, and my sentences broken into segments, and long words broken into syllables

—AND I learned to read and communicate well enough to be elected Governor of New York four times

—AND I won Congressional confirmation as Vice President of the United States

then I hope the telling of my story as a dyslexic will be an inspiration to the "puzzle children," for that is what I really care about. (Reprinted with permission from TV Guide® Magazine. Copyright © 1976 by Triangle Publications, Inc., Radnor, Pennsylvania.)

What was the key to Nelson Rockefeller's success in spite of being dyslexic? He was fiercely competitive. Instead of getting his feelings hurt when adults and roommates criticized him, he was determined to show them that he was just as smart as anyone else. This overachievement brought him all kinds of honors that did not seem possible for a dyslexic person. Rockefeller wanted to win badly enough to sacrifice pleasure, convenience, and comfort to reach his goals. The night he died of a heart attack, he was working on a publication that would share one of his main interests with the world. This dyslexic man would not give up.

Stephen J. Cannell

Not everyone has heard the name Stephen J. Cannell, but millions of people around the world have enjoyed the television programs "The Rockford Files," "Hardcastle and McCormick," "Riptide," and "The A-Team." The writer and producer of these highly successful television shows is dyslexic. Cannell remembers his dyslexic struggle getting through school. "When I was in junior high school," he recalls, "people used to say to me: 'Stephen, can't you look at that word and see it's not right?' But every time I looked at the word, it looked fine" (personal communication, 1988). There were times when this kind of pressure from teachers and friends would get him down. Sometimes he thought he could not do anything right. "Dyslexics tend to be pretty poor students," he remembers. "But it has nothing to do with intelligence. The biggest problem with dyslexic kids is that they get down on themselves. They can feel that they aren't smart in some ways, that they're retarded, and of course they aren't."

Cannell recalls that when he was growing up, dyslexia was still a mystery. No one understood it well enough to explain the problem to dyslexics themselves, or to parents and teachers. But Cannell decided to be a writer, even though he could not spell well or write without many mistakes. He developed strict habits for studying. He was up early every morning, not allowing himself to sleep late or to put off the task of getting to his work. In college he did a lot of writing. His professors would say: "Stephen, your writing is very interesting," but they would give him F because of poor spelling. Still, he knew that his ideas were good enough to put on paper. He developed a method of enrolling in college courses. He learned to ask each instructor: "What is your policy on misspellings?" He learned to find professors who would overlook poor spelling and give him credit for the value of his ideas and concepts. One professor became intrigued with his vivid storytelling ability and taught Cannell how to express his ideas in clear writing. This polished his visual imagination, which has produced some of the most popular television shows of the past decade.

Cannell is at work by 6:00 A.M. every day. He works steadily at his typewriter until 11:00 A.M. "My secretary has learned to figure out my mistakes," he explains. "What happens is that I tend to mirror-read and reverse letters. I am absolutely unaware that I am doing it. It slows me down as a reader and makes me a horrible speller because no word really looks right to me." In discussing his dyslexic problems publicly, Stephen hopes that he is a good role model for dyslexic youngsters. "I hope they are saying, 'Gee, here's a guy who couldn't even read and now he is making a living as a successful, famous writer.' "

How has Stephen Cannell overcome his dyslexic problems? He developed strong self-discipline, and learned to write at a keyboard. He learned to get his ideas onto paper though his keyboard, then let someone else worry about correct spelling, good grammar, and accurate punctuation. He learned not to feel sorry for himself. The key to his success is his ability to turn loose the worry and frustration of being dyslexic and let his mind soar with ideas. He allowed someone else to do the detail work of editing.

Phil Troyer

Few people have ever heard of Phil Troyer. Dyslexia almost destroyed his life before he found a source of love, acceptance, and guidance in overcoming his deep fear of failure. Troyer has recently published a novel (*Father Bede's Misfit*), a story about his own struggles to overcome his dyslexic handicap. Troyer was reared in a gentle Amish home, and his father was a college professor of English and dean of a well-known university. But it was considered weakness in his home for men to show emotion or affection. Phil was severely dyslexic, but his childhood problems were not diagnosed. His family had no idea why he struggled so hard yet achieved so little in academic learning. This deeply sensitive boy grew up without enough support to develop good self-esteem. He was a child during the 1940s before much was known about dyslexia. He vividly recalls the crushing experience he endured of being laughed at by classmates because he could not read, write, or spell. Adults were unsympathetic when he turned to parents and teachers for help. He grew up fearing that he was "dumb" and defective. He describes his teen years as "insecure, lonely, and frightening." There was no help available to relieve his misery.

In his early adult years, Troyer discovered a small monastery in New Mexico where he was taken in by the compassionate monks. Father Bede became especially interested in him and helped him become part of the monastic community. At the point of emotional breakdown, Phil began counseling with a psychiatrist who realized that he was dyslexic. This led to diagnosis of the problem. Phil began to write as part of his recovery therapy. Over a period of time he produced a manuscript that was published by York Press. The novel is a slightly fictionalized version of his life, telling the story of a dyslexic man who almost did not survive. Now that he is a published author, Troyer is finishing a second novel about his reconciliation with his father who learned to express his love for his son before his death.

How did Phil Troyer overcome dyslexia? When he was at the lowest possible level of depression and confusion, a loving counselor and mentor came into his life. This compassionate stranger soon became a strong friend who believed in Troyer at a time when he could not believe in himself. This unexpected demonstration of love and confidence awakened the life that had almost slipped away through despair. With the support of a loving community of dedicated friends, Phil Troyer came back to life. Through loving guidance and therapy he was able to rebuild his lost self-esteem and discover talent and intelligence within himself. With the help of others, he learned to overcome his dyslexic handicap.

Richard YaDeau

Richard YaDeau, MD, is a surgeon in St. Paul, Minnesota. He is also Director of Oncology at Bethesda Lutheran Medical Center in that city. In 1985 he became president of a nationwide nonprofit health maintenance organization that brings medical care to many people. He has guided the establishment of a hospice program in St. Paul where terminally ill patients may "die with dignity." Dr. YaDeau has vivid memories of being a dyslexic child, although his disability was not diagnosed until much later in his life. He failed his first 8 years in school. In spite of failing grades, he was "socially promoted" each year, entering each successive grade without the literacy skills to do the work. Then he was denied admission into high school until his father begged school administrators to give his son a chance. Later YaDeau would say: "It made me angry that school officials kept flunking me for spelling and would not listen to what I had to say." Eventually he was admitted to Yale University where he earned his undergraduate degree. Later he earned the MD degree from New York Medical College. He also served a successful tour of duty as an officer in the United States Marine Corps.

Like so many other "late blooming" dyslexics, YaDeau proved that he was capable of completing a complex education if officials would give him the opportunity. He will never forget how his parents were advised to enroll him in a trade school because it was believed he would never be able to handle college studies. He recalls being allowed to finish high school only because of his parents' constant pressure on school officials. Had school leaders had their way, he would have become an academic drop-out in his middle teens. What enabled Richard YaDeau to overcome dyslexia? His parents intervened on his behalf when no one else believed in him. Through their persistent pressure, school officials reluctantly gave him a chance, even though they were convinced it would be a waste of time. As he finished maturing during his late teens and early twenties, this late bloomer began to prove to skeptical adults that he had the potential for college success. Once he had earned his professional credentials, he proved himself worthy of his parents' trust. They believed in him when no one else would. For the past 25 years, Dr. Richard YaDeau has been an important influence in the St. Paul community.

Josef Sanders

One of the most courageous men I have ever known is Dr. Josef Sanders. He is dyslexic, yet he is the founder of a highly successful publishing company, Modern Education Corporation, which has delivered excellent educational materials for 20 years. He also is handicapped in reading and writing by dyslexia.

Like thousands of other dyslexic children in our culture, Joe Sanders was almost a casualty in his early years. He tells his story in the following words:

> I was LD before it was popular to be LD. I was born prematurely and weighed only 3 pounds, 2 ounces. In those days, it was tough dealing with premature babies. My development was fairly normal until it was time to begin to speak. I began to stutter at age 3 and continued stuttering until age 5. I used my left hand more than my right hand, and my parents were told to tie my left hand to my side to force me to be right-handed. My kindergarten teacher discovered that I had difficulty concentrating, and I talked a lot in class. I was never a discipline problem, but I was always restless in structured situations. I was told to wear glasses, but I hid them under my bed because I felt ugly wearing them. By the time I was in second grade, my learning problems were becoming obvious. I had difficulty learning to deal with symbols, both letters and numbers. My writing was very poor, and I had trouble following the teacher's directions. During second grade I realized that learning was becoming very difficult for me and that I was not catching on like my classmates. My teacher that year was frustrated with me. That was the first time I perceived myself as not being as good or as smart as other students. The teacher tied colored yarn on my wrists so I could tell the difference between right and left. I had great difficulty copying from the board. I severely reversed words (*was/saw, on/no*), and I had a hard time with *b, d,* and *p*. I could not write the alphabet without melody (singing the alphabet song).
>
> By the time I entered fourth grade, I was so far behind the others the principal called my parents in for a conference. They were told that

> I appeared to be mentally retarded, and they were advised to place me in a special school for mentally retarded children. I will never forget coming home from school and seeing my mother crying. I asked what was wrong, and she said that the principal had told her that I needed to go to Sunshine School. My first response was that it sounded like a nice place. Sunshine School sounded pleasant and pretty. I will never forget how this caused my mother to sob. Finally she told me that Sunshine School was for mentally retarded children. She explained that my school thought that I was mentally retarded and needed special education. The tone of my mother's voice struck fear into me. Suddenly I knew why she had been crying. All at once I realized that I was a different student. That moment was a major turning point in my life. I felt like a lost child with no sense of direction.
>
> A few days later, I discovered that I was a very fortunate person. My mother became intensely angry about what the principal had said. She vowed not to send me to that school for retarded children. She declared that she would work with me herself every day until I could read, write, spell, and do math like other kids my age. This was an awful, painful period for me and my family.
>
> As I struggled with my learning disabilities, I learned to escape from school frustration by playing by myself and using my imagination. I would create my own toys. My parents had very little money, and they could not buy things for me. So I created my own playthings. I learned to be grateful for being able to create things for myself. If I had the choice of playing or studying with my mother, I naturally chose to play outdoors. I did not like school and could not concentrate longer than a few minutes at a time. Half an hour of study with my mother was like an overweight 50-year-old man trying to run the Boston Marathon. It was difficult and very painful. My mind would wander, and I would cause my mother to become so frustrated. I just wanted to get out of the kitchen and play outdoors. Mother made me read aloud to her every day, and I hated it. Reading aloud is still a traumatic experience for me. I had so much trouble reading aloud in class or with my mother, I developed psychosomatic illnesses. The thought of reading aloud made me want to die. I could not breathe. My heart made palpitations. I was overwhelmed by extreme fear. My eyes could not track along the lines of the page. I stuttered and sounded like a little child just learning to read in first grade. I hated those times in reading circle or with my mother when I had to read aloud because my disability was always "found out." I sounded so dumb! To this day, all of those old feelings come back if I am asked to read aloud in public. Recently I turned down a prestigious part in a worship service at my synagogue because of this old phobia toward oral reading. (personal communication, 1988)

Josef Sanders struggled through high school and finally earned his diploma. Then he joined military service where he began to discover new skills within himself. Like most low birth weight boys, he was very late reaching important developmental milestones. He was a classic example of a late bloomer who began to blossom during his early twenties in military service. Eventually Sanders earned a bachelor's degree, then finally a doctorate in educational psychology. He earned his credential as a speech pathologist and worked for several years as a highly successful speech therapist. Then he entered private practice, working with frustrated youngsters who were struggling with learning disabilities. In the 1960s he founded Modern Education Corporation and began to market helpful materials for the field of special education.

What was the key to Sanders's success in overcoming dyslexia? It was his undying courage. No matter how difficult his life became through the pain of arthritis, the frustration of being dyslexic, and the anxiety of surviving the uncertain economics of private practice and running a business, he never gave up. His deep religious orientation has given him a sense of purpose, that he is on this earth for a reason, and that he will receive the strength he needs to function day to day. Sanders's courage has enabled him to overcome dyslexia.

How Do Successful Dyslexics Overcome Their Disabilities?

These examples of success by dyslexics contain a great deal of wisdom for those who struggle with learning disabilities. What does it take to deal successfully with the hidden handicap we call dyslexia? As we have seen in these brief glimpses into the lives of past and present dyslexics, certain factors must exist to enable frightened, frustrated, and even overwhelmed individuals to come to grips with their language disabilities. The following ingredients seem necessary to allow dyslexic strugglers to overcome their disabilities.

Anger

We must be careful to understand the role of anger in overcoming dyslexia. Of itself, anger is usually a destructive force that distorts reality and blocks the angry person's ability to deal with issues clearly. To be angry is to be deeply upset. To feel anger is to have adrenaline pour into the bloodstream to trigger the body's defenses against danger. To feel hot anger is to see an enemy who must be attacked and conquered. Anger is an explosion of the emotions.

This explosion usually destroys objective thinking at the moment and colors the intentions of others. To stay angry very long usually starts a chain reaction of destructive forces within one's body and personality. As a rule, we are wise to avoid being angry.

The kind of anger that helps dyslexics overcome their disabilities is in the form of righteous indignation. This can be a constructive emotion, being indignant over injustice. Indignation played a powerful role in Thomas Edison's victory. He would not accept the verdict that he was defective, retarded, or unworthy. His pride was wounded by his treatment by the schools of his day, and he vowed never to submit to that form of deprivation. Within this young man was a fiery indignation that smoldered like a carefully banked fire. He was angry to be treated in such a thoughtless fashion, and he simply would not permit it. This simmering resentment over the injustice of being wrongly labeled was the driving force that gave Edison the power to compensate and eventually overcome the disabling effects of dyslexia. Although his writing always contained poor spelling and limited language expression, he fiercely honed his skills to prove to the world that he was worthy of respect and admiration. Without this fire of anger, Edison, the right-brain genius, would never have emerged. Without the goading push of indignation, we would have lost this dyslexic man's vital contributions to our way of life. He had to become angry in order to survive. Fortunately, Thomas Edison had the devoted support of a mother who believed in her son and pledged with him to beat the odds. She forged the metal of his indignation into strategies of success. She helped him learn how to channel his anger, not waste his strength in useless battles against events and attitudes he could not change. She taught him how to use his angry strength to move the mountains that could be moved. With her help, he learned not to attack those mountains that could not be changed.

Edison's first motivation was to prove himself to a critical, skeptical world that did not care whether he lived or died. Unfortunately, many dyslexics find themselves undesirable and unattractive. Thomas Edison was rejected by his own father. He was pushed from the educational system of his day. He experienced failure at numerous jobs during his early years. He felt the hot surge of anger many times before age 20. But he learned how to turn this hostility and not allow it to devour his strength. Instead, he developed the ability to handle his indignation, molding it for his purposes instead of letting it consume him. This type of anger is essential for many dyslexics. It is often described as dyslexics tell their stories of success. Those who overcome this disability do not allow their anger to make them overly bitter or resentful. With age comes the wisdom to reflect on early struggles with the eye of the philosopher. An angry philosopher, to be sure, but not a bitter one. The right form of anger is one of the important keys to open the door to success after years of near-failure.

Pride

Like anger, pride is often the downfall of those who feel its intoxicating power. In its usual form, pride does indeed make tyrants and arrogant braggarts of us all. Raw pride is an ugly force that steps all over others and brags of its own worth. Unrefined pride struts and postures and claims rights it does not deserve to have. Basic human pride is regarded as sin by most religions. It is an emotion to be avoided, certainly not cultivated among our children. A proud person seldom is attractive. Pride is the root of all sorts of difficulties in human relationships. Of itself, pride is to be avoided and brought under control.

Yet pride is the key to success in many dyslexics. George S. Patton IV overcame his disabilities through pride. Perhaps he was not fully successful in taking the raw edge off his pride. History records many moments when he behaved in an arrogant fashion that disappointed his friends and created embarrassment for him. But Patton survived his reading disability because of his confidence in himself. When pride takes the form of self-confidence, it energizes the person to keep on trying. Pride must exist to a certain degree before a healthy self-image can develop. Being proud of oneself is essential before any person can develop the will to conquer the challenges ahead. Being sure of one's own worth is vital if any kind of victory over adversity is to be achieved. We must believe enough in ourselves to make the victory effort worthwhile. This is especially true for dyslexics.

As we listen to successful dyslexics tell their stories, we hear the quiet theme of pride underlying their achievements. It would be impossible for any person to conquer a language disability without a certain degree of pride. The struggling reader must feel worthy of learning to do difficult work better. Poor spellers must be discontent to have their personal worth so misrepresented. With today's electronic spelling help through word processors, this pride in achievement comes bursting into full view. Dyslexics who had to conquer the limitations of poor written language before spell-checkers were available had to be sure of their self-worth. Overcoming the disabling aspects of dyslexia requires pride in its positive form. In Chapter 6 we saw the unfortunate effects of arrogance and self-centeredness in the pathetic story of Joe. That kind of pride cannot help the dyslexic person break free. But a quiet, calm, low-key pride continually reassures the person: "I am worthy of success. I am worth what it costs to overcome this present condition. I have a worthwhile contribution to make in the years ahead. I am valuable. I am intelligent. I deserve an opportunity to prove myself." This is the voice of the kind of pride dyslexics must have before they can break the chains and overcome their childhood handicap.

Faith

Having faith is such a simple thing, yet it is not always found in those individuals who surround dyslexic children. Several of our success stories have included the element of faith. A mother believed in her child if other relatives did not. Parents believed when school leaders did not. The dyslexic person believed if all others did not. Faith is the most "blind" of all human emotions. Faith *knows* even when there is nothing tangible to see or provide a foundation for knowing. Faith is the most optimistic of all of our attitudes, because it insists that substance exists where only emptiness appears. Faith is composed of hope, and hope believes far beyond facts and solid data. Faith says that this struggling child is *not* retarded when test scores are within the retarded range. Faith looks beneath the surface of life and sees undeveloped potential that cannot be seen by casual observers. Faith sees random bits and pieces and immediately perceives a finished mosaic. Critics see only useless fragments that should be swept away. Faith looks at a deformed child and sees beauty in the soul and strength in the unbloomed intelligence. Faith does not give up when leadership wants to end the relationship and send the struggler away.

Faith, that invisible, rather foolish, unscientific, often irrational force is absolutely critical if strugglers are to overcome their struggles. Those of us who build our relationships upon faith continually hear suffering people say: "I could not have made it without you. You are the only one who still believes in me." Those of us who do intervention counseling with desperate people who reach the point of suicide often hear: "You are the only reason I am still alive. If it weren't for you, I would not be alive today." It is impossible for a child to survive the earlier years of dyslexic struggle without faith. Someone must believe in the child. Someone must be able to see beyond test scores or classroom behavior and recognize the potential that can be developed with patient care. Someone must teach the struggling dyslexic that he or she is worthy of being loved.

Someone must help that struggler recognize ways in which he or she has value and why that value must be preserved for the future. Someone must believe, or else there is no hope. Without hope, there is no reason to endure the almost endless conflicts that must be won if the dyslexic person is to overcome that difficulty. Faith is one of the most important keys to success for those who overcome dyslexia.

Inner Strength

Dyslexics who overcome their disabilities have an inner strength that does not always display itself on the surface. The stories about Woodrow Wilson and Albert Einstein tell of two language disabled men who at first seemed too weak to overcome their handicaps. They did not have the blustering self-confidence of George Patton. They did not display the fiery anger of young Thomas Edison. But as their lives slowly developed, those two men demonstrated enormous inner strength that allowed them to overcome their language disabilities. Wilson was able to become a successful speaker. He could convince world audiences of the merit of his concepts of peace. Einstein did not learn to speak or write fluently, but he manifested a relentless spirit that produced the revolutionary formula $E = MC^2$, which changed the course of human life forever. Dyslexics who overcome must have an inner strength that is as tough as an old oak tree whose roots anchor it firmly against hurricanes and tornadoes. These quiet ones must be able to absorb insult without breaking apart. They must be able to bend with the explosions around them, then come back to a standing position still upright and intact. One must have an inner structure as tough as iron if one is to live through the turmoil of growing up dyslexic, then overcome that pattern later on.

The quality of inner strength includes the ability to absorb enormous insult without retaliating. The teachings of Jesus include the fascinating concept of going the extra mile, doing more than is required, and surprising the adversary by unexpected acts of kindness. Dyslexics must often have this quality, this ability to absorb insult, this capacity to stand still in the face of powerful forces. It is impossible to overcome dyslexia if one insists upon fighting every battle that comes along. A certain degree of meekness must exist, the ability to turn the other cheek in the face of confrontation. During their quest to overcome their disabilities, dyslexics must be able to stop the urge to gain revenge. They must set aside the temptation of "an eye for an eye, a tooth for a tooth." Learning disabled persons who react to conflict on that level usually do not overcome their problems successfully. Overcoming dyslexia requires enough quiet inner strength to absorb hostility without blowing it out of proportion.

Competitive Spirit

As we have seen in the stories of Albert Einstein and Woodrow Wilson, not all dyslexics succeed through competition. Dr. Josef Sanders did not need to defeat his critics in order to climb to the top of his profession. But certain individuals like Nelson Rockefeller do find their victory through competition. The urge to compete is the key that opens the future to certain persons. There is a heady quality in competition. The challenge of winning triggers the adrenaline flow that kicks the person's skills into overdrive. Those who have the competitive spirit are lost when there is no challenge. They do not develop interest unless there is a clearly defined adversary to overcome. This spirit of competition can easily get out of control, of course. We all recoil from fiercely competitive people who thrive on challenge. Overly aggressive people who live for competition are very uncomfortable to be with. Like prancing, high-spirited colts in a stockade, it is not safe to be in their presence. But the competitive spirit that enables dyslexics to overcome is a more disciplined attitude. They respond to the gauntlet, of course, but they do not intend to hurt or deprive others as they achieve their goals. Being competitive is often the key that certain dyslexics need to achieve success.

As adults like Nelson Rockefeller tell their stories, we hear an underlying theme of thoughtfulness and concern for others. In Chapter 6 we pondered the unfortunate pattern called social disability. This includes self-centeredness, which is a universally unpleasant characteristic in others. The competitive spirit described in Rockefeller's account is a compassionate attitude, not an aggressive desire to dominate. Persons like Rockefeller need the challenge of someone like his roommate Johnny. The spirit of competition cannot see itself except by looking into the mirror of challenge. Once competitiveness sees its counterpart in the mirror, it is able to focus energy toward specific, well-defined goals. Without this focus through challenge, dyslexics like Rockefeller do not have clear enough vision to know how to move ahead successfully. As we have seen, certain individuals like Albert Einstein are able to see themselves clearly without standing before the mirror of challenge. If so, then the spirit of competition is not part of their way to success. But the competitive spirit is essential for certain people who cannot define themselves any other way.

Self-Discipline

Every dyslexic who overcomes must be self-disciplined. This is the glue that holds all other ingredients of success together. As we have seen in several of our success stories, each person must learn how to say no to things that would distract them from their main goals. Everyone who succeeds must be able to start early, as Rockefeller and Cannell explained, instead of sleeping in and taking it easy. Those dyslexics who succeed must be able to ignore pain, inconvenience, disappointment, frustration, depression, and all of the other voices that whisper continually for attention. Being self-disciplined is being able to make one's own plans, manage one's own time, meet one's own obligations on schedule, control desires that would eat up scarce resources, and so forth. Dyslexics must develop skills in disciplining themselves, or else they cannot overcome their handicaps.

Cultivating self-discipline is probably the least appealing activity anyone is asked to do. If human characteristics were given colors, self-discipline would probably be dull gray. Staying in control of self is a parental role. One cannot romp as a carefree youngster and be self-disciplined. One cannot always take second helpings or have rich desserts or satisfy strong cravings the moment they arise. Self-discipline is like a parent having to say no to a clamoring child. Staying in charge of oneself is not always a pleasant activity. When everyone else is goofing off or out at the lake or on a holiday, self-discipline sternly says: "No, you have to stay home and work." Everyone gets tired of doing one's duty. Everyone wants to take a break at some point. The self-disciplined person must do duty and keep on with chores until important things are accomplished.

As Nelson Rockefeller so clearly explained, self-discipline is the structure that holds the dyslexic pieces firmly in place. When the loose pieces of dyslexia are carefully organized into a solid mosaic, self-discipline is the glue that makes the picture stay together. Dyslexics who fail are those who never develop the structure of self-discipline. They go through life with too many pieces missing from their mosaic. Those who overcome are the ones who learn how to say no to some of the ways the self clamors for satisfaction.

Loving Support

No one has yet researched the effect of love upon the lives of dyslexics, but it does not require validated studies to know that love is an essential key. The story of Phil Troyer brings our attention quickly to this vital fact. As we have seen in Chapter 5, love was missing from the life of Shane, the boy who was so defeated by guilt. Through the years, I have known many dyslexics who did not have enough loving support to sustain them. Those of us who counsel dyslexics of all ages deal continually with devastating emotions that destroy self-esteem when the suffering person has no one to whom he or she can turn for love and reassurance. Every dyslexic success story is about loving support from some important source. I am always shocked to hear a sorrowing dyslexic person say: "You are the only one who still loves me after the mess I've made of everything." When loving support is taken away by those who lose faith, there is often nothing left upon which the dyslexic person can depend. Many attempts at suicide are triggered when the struggling person realizes that no one cares.

As we look at the ingredients and keys to success in the stories we hear from victorious dyslexics, we always hear about loving support. This support usually comes more from mothers than it comes from fathers. During the past 30 years, I have seen many grandparents assume this role of loving support. Often we see an uncle or aunt do so. Youngsters often find loving support within their extended families of religious leaders, scout leaders, and teachers. Dyslexic teenagers often form their own support groups, finding among their peers the nonjudgmental acceptance they cannot find elsewhere. I have seen caring support behind prison walls where we least expect to find it. We often see a kind of loving support within military units where men and women live in close quarters. Dyslexic students who succeed in adult education find support, or they do not succeed. It is impossible to overcome dyslexia if one is all alone.

As we have seen in several stories, the presence of loving support is a healing agent for the embattled child. To spend a day struggling through school, as Josef Sanders described, is to suffer emotional bruises and wounds. To be a dyslexic within a high-achieving family often inflicts battle scars upon the ego structure of the vulnerable child. To be dyslexic in a competitive world where everyone else earns praise is to expose oneself to constant danger of emotional injury. The vulnerable child must have a source of healing from day to day. Loving support is the healing medicine for these battle-weary strugglers.

A Friendly Advocate

Every dyslexic must have someone on his or her side. This goes beyond the loving support we have just described. There must also be someone to play the role of attorney, someone to speak out on the struggler's behalf, someone to argue his or her case when words fail. Someone must be there who believes, who cares, and who will come to the dyslexic person's defense. This is usually the mother. When matters become serious, many fathers step in for a while. Teachers frequently intervene on the behalf of a struggling student. School counselors are forever trying to change a teacher's mind regarding a low-achieving student. Dyslexics are often able to go long periods of time managing fairly well if their lives are well structured. But at some point, every dyslexic person must have a friendly advocate to speak for him or her or present a defense.

As I look back over the past quarter century of working with dyslexics, I see many who failed. In almost every case, there was no friendly advocate to intervene, and the language disabled person lost the battle. He or she could not find the words to defend against articulate, aggressive authority. Occasionally we see stubbornness in a dyslexic person, as Chapter 6 explains. Stubbornness can defeat the efforts of friendly advocates. But in most instances, dyslexic failure occurs when there is no one to take the side of the struggler. Conversely, all dyslexic persons I have seen succeed had a friendly advocate, someone who took their case and defended them when intervention was necessary. Dr. Sanders and Dr. YaDeau tell of their advocates who took charge of their troubles and guided them safely through. In both stories, it was parents who played that role. Having a friendly advocate to speak on one's behalf is of critical importance if dyslexics are to overcome.

Courage

I have been astonished many times over the level of courage I have seen in struggling learners. I have needed a certain degree of courage in my own life, but I have never faced the enormous problems day after day that dyslexics in our culture face. It is impossible to survive dyslexia in the Western world without courage. As children struggle through their school years, they often do not realize that their level of struggle is unusual. They often assume that everyone has to work just as hard. These naive ones are usually amazed when they learn that their classroom struggle is actually unique among their peers. How can a rational person face certain failure day after day without becoming mentally ill? How can children who have learning disabilities endure the constant threat of failure and disappointment without at least becoming neurotic? How do dyslexics who cannot read, write, spell, or do math computation adequately survive mainstream education where busy teachers often have no idea how to meet their needs? This kind of life requires enormous courage. The dyslexics who succeed do indeed exhibit the courage and emotional toughness to face daily failure without becoming neurotic or mentally ill. Those who do not possess enough courage go under. The Menninger Foundation has begun to map certain forms of mental illness that emerge within the dyslexic population during middle teens (Jernigan, 1985). It is not yet clear what relationship dyslexia actually has with this suffering population. However, it is known that eating disorders (anorexia nervosa and bulimia) appear more often within the learning disabled population than among students who have no learning disorders. Certain forms of adolescent schizophrenia also appear to occur more frequently among our struggling learners.

The point is that being learning disabled in today's educational environment requires a great deal of courage. How does a child face the stigma of being called "lazy?" When the important adults in the child's life insist: "You're just not trying hard enough. You could do better if you tried harder," what does the child do? When smart-aleck remarks are made by peers about "going to the dummy class" as the child goes down the hall for special help, what does the struggling learner do? When an inflexible or incompetent psychometrist reports a low IQ score on a timed, standardized test, how does the dyslexic child handle the shocking conclusion that he or she is "moderately retarded?" When classmates win praise and have their better work displayed, how does the embarrassed dysgraphic child cope with his or her "messy" papers? When everyone else is telling stories about academic victories, what does the struggling learner say? To survive 12 or 13 years in such an environment should produce several million mentally disturbed children. Yet it does not. How do these disabled learners survive? They survive because they have courage. They have a built-in toughness that enables them to deal with chronic near-failure successfully. Not happily. Not joyfully. Often with much pain. But if they have courage, they make it through those destructive years with only old scars left to show their conflict.

No Self-Pity

A dyslexic cannot overcome if he or she wallows in self-pity. As we have heard in several of our success stories, self-pity cannot be part of the victory celebration. To feel sorry for self is to turn inward. "Poor little me! Look at my misfortune! Life is not fair! Everyone else is to blame! Look, everyone, look at me! Poor, pitiful little me!" That cannot be within the vocabulary of dyslexic persons if they are to overcome their disability patterns. Self-pity is an ugly characteristic in any person. As we saw in Chapter 6, feeling sorry for oneself cripples the personality so that no strength is left for forward movement. Self-pity drains away vital emotional energy that is needed to sustain courage. Wallowing in the dark pool of self-pity submerges the person in a sticky emotional mess that quickly snuffs out any beauty that person may have. No one has much sympathy for someone who shows self-pity. This is especially true for learning disabled strugglers.

The antidote for self-pity is a sense of humor, at least to some degree. No one can laugh very much at true misfortune. There is nothing to chuckle over when one is in pain. But the attitude of humor must flourish strongly enough to enable the struggler to break free when self-pity reaches out to take control. As we have seen in earlier chapters, parents and teachers must begin early in the dyslexic child's life to teach the survival skill of avoiding the clutches of self-pity. When self-pity reaches out to grip one's emotions, each of us must have the strength to push it away. It is impossible to overcome dyslexia if self-pity is an active part of one's life.

8

Looking to the Future for Dyslexics

When I began working with the dyslexic population in the late 1950s, the word *dyslexia* was not included in most dictionaries. Only a few professionals and educators had heard the term, and it was generally regarded with skepticism and disbelief. During my years as college professor, including my tenure as department chairman at a major university, my research with dyslexic students was often ridiculed by colleagues who were embarrassed to have that kind of irregular study conducted by their school.

This skeptical attitude toward dyslexia has begun to change. During the 1980s dyslexia has become the most thoroughly researched area of specific learning disability (Duane, 1985, 1987). More scientific data now exist confirming dyslexia than regarding any other form of learning dysfunction. Groups like the Orton Dyslexia Society and Association for Children and Adults with Learning Disability (ACLD) have sponsored in-depth research by leading scientists into the causes of dyslexia. Internationally recognized researchers such as Norman Geschwind, Albert Galaburda, Antonio Damasio, William Deering, Jane Flynn, Drake Duane, Sondra Jernigan, Veronika Grimm, and others have been mapping the geography of the brain. They have shown us where dyslexia occurs within the left and right brain hemispheres. Any professional today who disbelieves the existence of dyslexia or ridicules the issue is embarrassingly obsolete. It is no longer possible for educators, physicians, or counselors to toss dyslexia aside as just a notion. While we are still in the pioneering stage of fully understanding this problem, there is no longer lack of evidence that it does exist.

Our growing knowledge of brain-based learning dysfunctions, especially dyslexia, is pointing the way toward a hopeful future for dyslexics. My career in dealing with this problem has consisted mostly of educated guesses and shrewd hunches. The techniques my generation used with this special population from the 1950s to the late 1970s were largely trial and error. Certain teaching strategies worked well in establishing left-to-right sequence and overcoming reversals, but we did not have a truly scientific foundation for what we did. For example, in the 1940s Grace Fernald pioneered the technique of using sand trays and cut-out sandpaper for finger tracing of letters and words. Beth Slingerland developed the diagnostic strategies that became the highly successful Slingerland Screening Tests for Identifying Children with Specific Language Disabilities. Anna Gillingham collaborated with the late Dr. Samuel Orton to develop the Orton/Gillingham method for teaching literacy skills to dyslexics of all ages. But we did not have much scientific evidence to back our theories. As we look forward, we can give much more solidly based hope to future generations of dyslexic students.

Early Identification

As we have seen in Chapter 6, it is of critical importance that dyslexia be identified early so that effective teaching and counseling strategies can be started to offset the crushing impact of school failure. In the late 1980s several long-term studies were being concluded that have followed groups of dyslexics over long periods of time. For example, Dr. Mary Lee Enfield (1987) has concluded a 19-year study of dyslexic students in the Bloomington, Minnesota, public schools. In the 1960s she and her colleagues designed an intervention program based upon Samuel Orton's "three musts" for successful remediation of dyslexia: (1) direct instruction, (2) systematic phonics, and (3) multisensory rehearsal as the child learns. Enfield and her colleagues have documented that this basic approach works well with the dyslexic population. Classroom teachers are taught how to deal with these irregular learners within the mainstream classroom program instead of sending them down the hall for special work in an isolated resource room. The Bloomington, Minnesota, program has been so successful that it has been adopted by many schools in the United States. This mainstream approach to teaching dyslexics will be part of the future. There are two keys to its success: (1) teaching classroom teachers how to work effectively with dyslexic students, and (2) identifying specific language problems early enough in the child's school experience so that self-image is not damaged through too much failure.

Another pioneer in early identification of language disabilities is Dr. Barbara Wilson, chief of the Division of Neuropsychology, North Shore University Hospital, Manhasset, New York (Wilson & Risucci, 1988). Wilson and her colleagues have followed several groups of youngsters long enough to pinpoint predictive factors in the way certain children struggle with early language development. Wilson and her associates are now defining an early childhood language pattern called Delayed Language Development (DLD) Syndrome. By spotting certain language deficits by age 4, it is possible to predict which children will have dyslexic struggles later when they encounter reading, spelling, and writing instruction. Wilson's research has yielded the following list of behaviors to look for in young children who are just learning to talk:

1. Poor hearing
2. Atypical (irregular) language development
3. Poor auditory perception (inability to keep up in listening)
4. Poor auditory cognition (inability to understand what is heard)
5. Poor short-term memory
6. Poor organizational ability
7. Poor naming
8. Poor word retrieval (inability to remember words learned earlier)
9. Poor visual discrimination
10. Poor spatial perception
11. Poor visual cognition (inability to interpret what is seen)
12. Poor response to instructions
13. Poor expressive language ability

In the future, adults who work with toddlers and preschool children will have this kind of diagnostic guideline to help them spot dyslexia even before children start to school. Early recognition of language problems will help future teachers get to work early enough with dyslexic children to avoid the tragic losses so many dyslexics have experienced in the past (Rees, 1978).

Brain Scan Information

As brain scan techniques become more sophisticated, it will become routine to check the central nervous system of children, adolescents, and adults in ways that pose no threat to the person's health (Shucard, Cummins, Gay, Lairsmith, & Welanko, 1985). By the mid-1980s several "nonintrusive" brain scan systems were available. For example, evoked potential EEG stimulates several areas of the brain and records irregular patterns for detailed study. This is a safe way to study brain wave patterns, and it often reveals dyslexic tendencies within the left cerebral cortex. Most larger communities have the ability to perform CAT scans. This computer-based technique "photographs" the interior of the body from all angles. The CAT scan procedure is successful in spotting differences and abnormalities in all organs of the body. The CAT scan technique often helps to determine if the brain structure is normal or abnormal.

Several new brain scan systems are showing great promise for giving specific information about how brains function. One technique is called PET scan. This method uses tiny amounts of radioactive isotopes to make brain centers "glow." The PET scanner then photographs different brain centers as they work. It is possible to compare nondyslexic brains with dyslexic brains doing such work as reading, spelling, listening, writing, and speaking. PET scan results can pinpoint dyslexic-like brain structure, which helps to explain why certain students struggle with left-brain learning. Another body scan technique is based upon magnetic resonance (MRI). This shows the interior of the body in great detail. MRI scans produce detailed images of the brain, pinpointing abnormalities and differences in brain structure. The MRI technique shows much promise for spotting neuronal differences related to learning disability. Still another brain scan method, called BEAM, has the ability to trigger specific activity within various parts of the brain. By exciting specific brain areas for very brief moments (one one-thousandth of a second), it is possible to evoke a variety of responses such as Surprise Wave, Recognition Wave, Selective Attention Wave, Sexual Orientation Wave. This kind of research will eventually allow researchers to map brain abilities in great detail. Researchers believe that by the early 21st century, we will have the ability to map learning disability brain waves to guide us in teaching dyslexic children the most effective way. These and other research methods will open vast areas of knowledge into how the living brain functions or fails to function normally (Coppola, 1985).

As we listen to researchers discuss these kinds of new technologies, it is exciting to realize that within two or three decades, it will be possible to identify dyslexic brains very early, even before a child is born. Pioneers of fetal development such as Bruce McEwen (1986) of the Rockefeller University School of Medicine and Veronika Grimm (1986) of the Weizmann Institute of Science in Israel predict routine prenatal tests for dyslexia, the way we now test developing fetuses for Down's Syndrome and other genetic deficits. This kind of knowledge always holds double power, of course. In the wrong hands, it can become a tool of evil, used to "weed out" undesirable characteristics within our culture. There is always the risk of evil when we acquire new knowledge. Any good can potentially be used for harmful purposes. However, the hope for future treatment of dyslexia is that detection of the pattern during fetal development will allow us to begin remedial steps early enough to avoid heartbreak later on. The great heartache of dyslexia has been to discover it by accident after the child's self-esteem has been shattered through failure. In the past, treating dyslexia has often begun too late to avoid deep scars and loss of potential. In the future, detecting dyslexia in the developing fetus would allow parents to prepare for effective remedial steps in language development techniques from the time of infancy. We know that the earlier dyslexia is identified, the more effectively it can be remediated. Future diagnosis of dyslexia will include discovering it before the child is born.

Improved Physical Health of Dyslexics

A great deal of attention has been focused by researchers upon health patterns of dyslexics and their relatives. During their studies of dyslexics through the Harvard Medical School, Norman Geschwind and his colleagues gathered much information about the relatives of dyslexics (Geschwind, 1983, 1985). Before his untimely death in 1984, Dr. Geschwind published a summary of the health patterns his team had mapped in the families of dyslexics. There is a much higher than average number of left-handed persons within the genetic lines of dyslexics. There is a tendency for relatives to turn gray or become white-haired in their twenties or early thirties. Relatives of dyslexics tend to have overly sensitive digestive tracts with chronic problems related to how the body processes foods and beverages. Within family patterns of dyslexics, there is a higher than normal tendency for stomach ulcers, duodenal ulcers, colitis, and chronic bowel problems such as Crohn's Disease. Relatives of dyslexics have a higher than normal occurrence of autoimmune disorders. This refers to the tendency of the body to fight itself through such illnesses as lupus and arthritis. Autoimmune disorders include deficits in basal metabolism, the endocrine system, and thyroid production, which cause the body to make itself ill. Relatives of dyslexics have much higher than normal levels of chronic allergies, including asthma and respiratory problems. This leaves the person open to infection that leads to frequent bronchitis and pneumonia. Families of dyslexics also tend to overreact to specific food substances that cause cytotoxic problems. Researchers (Hagerman, 1983; Philpott, 1978; Wunderlich, 1978) have shown that there is a higher than normal level of hyperactivity among relatives of dyslexics, and there is higher than normal need to eliminate specific things from the diet, such as refined sugar, white wheat products, grape extracts and derivatives, salicylic foods (green peppers, strawberries), and chemical additives such as dyes and preservatives. It is clearly seen that families of dyslexics tend to have more health-related problems than the rest of the population (Cott, 1978).

As this kind of information becomes more generally known by pediatricians, parents, counselors, and educators, dyslexics in the future will receive more specific health care. Parents will be counseled from the beginning that the health of the dyslexic child will likely need extra attention. Cytotoxic reaction to culprit foods and beverages can be avoided by eliminating certain substances from the diet. The tendency for chronic allergies will be treated early enough to avoid years of health struggle and not feeling well, which directly interferes with classroom learning. Short attention span can be lengthened significantly by controlling problems within the body that keep the child's attention distracted from learning. Dyslexic children of the future will not need to endure years of physical discomfort and distraction before their health needs are recognized. Pediatricians of the 21st century will be educated in how to supervise the special health needs of this special population.

Improved Mental Health of Dyslexics

For the past 30 years I have been closely involved with hundreds of dyslexic youngsters as they have progressed from childhood through adolescence into adulthood. Those of us who have had this kind of long-range involvement with dyslexia have seen a great deal of anguish, frustration, and inability to cope with life on an emotional or spiritual level. During the 1980s several researchers have begun to map the mental health patterns of dyslexia and other forms of learning disability. For example, the Menninger Foundation in Topeka, Kansas, was among the first mental health institutions to recognize the fragile ego strength of many dyslexic youngsters (Jernigan, 1985). Psychiatrists and psychologists at the Menninger Foundation have studied mental health tendencies within the dyslexic population treated at that institution. For several years, all new patients entering the Menninger Clinic for psychotherapy have been screened for dyslexia. Dr. Sondra Jernigan has developed sophisticated evoked potential EEG evaluation techniques to identify "deep dyslexia" or primary dyslexia in new patients.

These kinds of studies have found that a certain number of dyslexic youngsters will develop mental health problems as they enter puberty. It is now seen that eating disorders (anorexia nervosa and bulimia) occur much more often among dyslexic teenagers than among the nondyslexic population. We now realize that certain forms of psychotic illness also emerge as certain dyslexic youngsters reach their middle teens. These psychotic breaks with reality often begin to diminish and even disappear by the early twenties. We now see that certain dyslexics will go through a "twilight zone" of mental illness that stretches from about age 15 to about age 25. Dyslexics are much more likely to suffer chronic depression and manic/depressive illness than the nondyslexic population. These new insights are still in infant stages of research. It is too early to predict which youngsters are at risk for mental health problems, or which young people are vulnerable to eating disorder. Yet the insights already gained show us hopeful expectation for the future.

At some point during the 21st century we will understand enough about the mental health needs of dyslexics to be able to predict which children will need mental health intervention. We already have a wide variety of medications to control several forms of schizophrenia, manic/depressive illness, paranoia, and the panic-attack suffering of certain individuals. Further research will produce medications to help offset the problems of social disability, Dyslogic Syndrome, and Right Hemi Syndrome, which were described in Chapter 6. While medication should never be used merely to repress emotional problems, the anguish that many dyslexics suffer can be reduced through thoughtful medication. As Bruce McEwen stated in 1986: "There is no such thing as a purely psychological process. Everything is at least partly related to body processes." This concept of mental health care will release dyslexics of the future from unnecessary years of anguish and defeat. When the body processes cause abnormalities in emotions and mental health, then appropriate medical intervention is required. Dyslexics who grow up in the 21st century will have access to sophisticated help through medication with wise supervision.

Improved Counseling and Guidance

A major change of direction in psychotherapy occurred during the 1970s with the emergence of Ecological Psychiatry (Ochroch, 1981; Philpott, 1978; Slavin, 1978). As new discoveries were made related to brain functions and how body processes do indeed influence mental health, more and more psychiatrists and psychologists began to view mental health through the lens of physical well being. How the patient's body functions determines to a large extent how the patient can interact with his or her world. There now exists substantial professional interest in physical health as it relates to mental health. Ecological psychiatry looks first at the body processes when a breakdown in mental health occurs. Detailed analysis is done of basal metabolism to find any irregularity in body chemistry functions. The patient's diet and eating habits are closely studied. Patterns of rest and fatigue are analyzed. The therapist examines the patient's life-style carefully for sources of stress or abuse. Ecological psychiatry proceeds from the point of view that we cannot improve mental health until interfering body processes are corrected. Once the body is functioning normally, then steps can be taken to improve mental health.

This approach to counseling and guidance has deep implications for the future treatment of dyslexia. Those of us who have guided many dyslexics to success have had to deal with body processes. They cannot be ignored. Having problems with one's body is directly distracting for anyone. Trying to overcome one's dyslexic problems if one's body is not well compounds the struggle intensely.

In the years ahead the physical needs of the dyslexic will be recognized by most counselors. Mental health professionals of the future will know much more about how dyslexics tend to be different in important physical ways. We have known for years that traditional counseling (talking over problems and pledging to change how one behaves) has little effect upon dyslexic behavior. Now we know why. The brain structures are different in dyslexic students. Body chemistry is often out of balance, which sets off chain reactions that soon make it impossible for the person to control emotions or concentrate well enough to learn. Control of impulses is often deficient, leaving the dyslexic person unable to stop a surge of anger or say no to a sudden rush of desire. Traditional counseling cannot change these body-based patterns unless the physical problems are treated first. Then the dyslexic person can begin to learn new habits through counseling. This will be the perspective of counseling with dyslexics in the future.

Preparation of Teachers

For many years we have faced a dilemma in preparing teachers. How do professors of education pass on new knowledge to future teachers when those professors have been isolated from the world of classroom learning? The greatest challenge of preparing future teachers is making sure that professors of education keep abreast of the latest knowledge related to classroom learning. Of all professions, it is essential that those who teach future teachers be at the leading edge of knowledge themselves. This has been especially true in the area of dyslexia. Few professors of education had any firsthand experience in dealing with dyslexia when they were classroom teachers themselves. Few of them learned up-to-date knowledge of dyslexia during their own graduate studies. If dyslexia was studied at all, it was often handled briefly as part of a larger unit of study about learning disabilities of all types. Moreover, as late as the mid-1980s, most professors of education tended to dismiss the "notion" of dyslexia as either unimportant or as a concept to be avoided by future teachers. It goes without saying that teachers teach what they know to teach. Preparing new teachers obviously depends upon the knowledge and experience of those in charge of the preparation. If one's professors do not know, or if they actively oppose certain concepts, then teachers in training either will not know or they will carry professors' negative attitudes into the classrooms of the future.

There has always been a very slow trickle-down tendency in teacher preparation. As a rule, it takes approximately 15 years for important new research discoveries to become a standard part of teacher education. Exciting, relevant, highly significant findings about how certain students learn will not be commonly disseminated within professional circles for 3 to 5 years following the discovery. As this new information appears in influential professional journals, it gradually becomes incorporated into new textbook chapters being written for publication. It usually requires 3 to 5 years for a new textbook to reach the reading public. Then there is the slow process of schools of education adopting new textbooks for future teachers to study. As this slow publication process takes place, alert instructors begin to include new concepts in their oral presentations, such as seminars, keynote speeches at conventions, and workshops. The oral tradition moves faster than the printed tradition. By the time important new information about a specific issue becomes widely incorporated into the preparation of teachers, it is often obsolete. It is incredibly difficult for teacher education to keep abreast of important new information when traditional dissemination routes are followed.

Fortunately, the preparation of teachers for the 21st century will be improved. Already a strong move is under way to upgrade requirements for those who will be the teachers of tomorrow. Within the next decade most colleges of education will require higher admissions standards, ensuring that only bright, capable young adults will be admitted to teacher training programs. Several states already require an internship that must be completed successfully before a teaching credential is issued. This means that after 4 or 5 years of college study, the prospective teacher must successfully finish 1 or 2 years of classroom instruction under the supervision of experienced teachers. While this internship approach will not guarantee that new teachers will know how to deal with dyslexia successfully, moving teacher preparation from the college campus into the laboratory of actual school classrooms will greatly increase exposure to struggling students who need special help with learning.

Teacher preparation for the future will respond to parental pressures more than in the past. Two well-organized professional parent/professional groups are pressing elected officials on all levels to give special consideration to learning disabled students. The Orton Dyslexia Society and the Association for Children and Adults with Learning Disability (ACLD) are highly effective lobby groups, influencing legislators to upgrade laws regarding the education of children with special needs.

Most of the progress in educating learning disabled students has come through the efforts of these two parent/professional organizations. A great deal more political activity on behalf of dyslexic students will be seen in years ahead. Preparation of teachers will be closely monitored to make sure that new teachers are adequately prepared to meet the needs of special students. Models like Dr. Enfield's program in Bloomington, Minnesota, will become the standards of teacher preparation for the 21st century. A major goal will be to cut the trickle-down time in half, enabling new teachers to receive new knowledge twice as soon as we have seen in the past.

New Technology

Anyone who studied math before 1965 used a slide rule. By 1970 the pocket calculator was within the price range of every student, and the slide rule suddenly became a museum piece. Today only older generations remember how to do math with that odd-looking device. A similar revolution is occurring in the 1980s in the area of writing, spelling, and editing. The word processor is rapidly replacing traditional handwriting and typing. It is ironic that the only place where handwriting is still the standard form of written expression is in the school classroom. Again, slow trickle-down tendencies make education obsolete. It is rare to find an elementary school or middle school math program where hand calculators are permitted. Math students still slave over memorizing arithmetic facts and hours of homework with pencil processing. However, in the school office, every form of number work is done with calculators and computers. Back in the classroom, pupils must still toil with obsolete handwritten methods until they reach high school math, where calculators are introduced as a welcome tool. The same story can be told about word processors. Thousands of microcomputers sit in classrooms while students toil away with pencils and ballpoint pens. Outsiders often have the impression that educators still have not entered the 20th century, which is about to end, when it comes to teaching students to use new technology.

It would be hard to find a child who is not a whiz with some kind of electronic video game. Preschoolers spend a lot of time with battery-operated toys that beep and blink and whistle and do all sorts of things electronically. Every Christmas season brings a wave of new electronic gadgets that are immediately absorbed into childhood lifestyles. Adults are often irritated by ever-present video games that intrude noisily everywhere. Youngsters are almost universally fluent and comfortable with this new world of electronic pleasure. Children with severe left-brain disabilities in reading and language usage usually have no difficulty with the right-brain skills of video games and electronic devices.

The future holds great promise for dyslexics through new electronic technology (Boettcher, 1983; Steeves, 1987). The educational problem of dyslexics is their inability to do left-brain language-based activities well. But the right brain is seldom learning disabled or dyslexic. The electronic world is a right-brain world, and this is home territory for most dyslexics. This is why few dyslexic children have trouble learning to type, then learning to work with a microcomputer or a word processor. Those who struggle hard to write legibly or to spell correctly have little difficulty learning to tap out information on a keyboard, then interpret it from a screen. This technology provides an excellent bridge between left-brain requirements and right-brain processing. Tapping out information on a keyboard is mostly a right-brain function, which lets left-brain dyslexics bypass or compensate for their academic struggles. Future generations of dyslexics will be able to bypass their learning disabilities almost entirely, once classroom education catches up with 20th century progress. This will occur rapidly as younger teachers who have grown up in an electronic world replace older educators who often are computer-illiterate.

During the 1980s a wide variety of microcomputer systems appeared. The technology of self-editing became available to children. Most of the home computer systems purchased by parents have included some kind of spell-checker program that searches the typed document for spelling errors. One of the first student-oriented spell-check systems was the Bank Street Speller designed mostly for Apple II computers. Many educators discovered that once dyslexic students were taught to operate these units correctly, they began pouring out reams of intelligent written material. Several research projects have demonstrated an astonishing growth in the writing of dyslexics. For example, Dr. Joyce Steeves (1987), Research Associate at the Johns Hopkins University School of Education, found that dyslexic boys tend to write 15 sentences on the computer/word processor for every sentence they write with a pencil. Teachers who have incorporated computer/word processor writing into classroom language skill development are astonished to see the greatly increased fluency of writing, especially by students who struggle to produce meager written work with a pencil. Keyboard writing is clearly the technology of the future for dyslexics.

It is impossible for anyone to keep track of all the new microcomputer technology. Manufacturers of home computers are in fierce competition to produce upgraded systems and programs. By the late 1980s highly sophisticated spell-checker programs were available at low cost, such as Webster's New World Spelling Checker (Simon and Schuster, Inc.), or Wordstar Professional, Release 4 (Micropro International Corporation). With careful training in using these systems, most dyslexics can find and correct 70% of their own spelling errors. By the year 2000 dyslexics will also have self-editing software programs that will find mistakes in grammar and punctuation. Before the turn of this century, dyslexic students will have lap-size computers available at low cost. These personal computers can be carried to class, set on a small desk top, and used to write themes, reports, or test responses in class. These compact units will include spell-check programs, as well as programs to edit punctuation, capitalization, and grammar. These portable word processors will do for writing what the pocket calculator did for math. Within the near future, traditional pencil writing will become obsolete as our culture adapts to new writing technologies. In the future dyslexics will be able to compete successfully with nondyslexics through "writing calculators."

Still another form of electronic editor is rapidly becoming available for the dyslexic population. Small, pocket-size spelling checkers are already on the market. For example, in 1987 the Impact Merchandising Corporation of San Ramon, California, introduced a revolutionary compact spell-checker. The Franklin Spelling Ace weighs 8 ounces and fits into a large pocket. It has a small standard keyboard with a small display screen. The memory system contains 80,000 commonly used words, as well as extra memory capacity for individualized word lists which students may want to develop. By typing a word on the keyboard, the student can check any spelling within the memory bank. The Franklin Spelling Ace uses state-of-the-art spelling clues to find misspellings that often barely resemble the correct word. In competitive tests, this personal "spelling calculator" has outperformed most of the more expensive microcomputer spell-check programs. Now the dyslexic student has a small battery-operated "spelling calculator" that can fit inside a notebook, book bag, or coat pocket. Using this kind of electronic helper will still be slow, but it will give poor spellers an ever-present editor for writing that must be done in class. Within a few years this kind of help will be available for only a few dollars to every student, the way pocket calculators became available by 1970.

Still another electronic writing device to help future dyslexics is the voice writer. The first commercial models of the voice writer will appear soon. As technology improves, voice writers will become sophisticated and inexpensive. The voice writer listens to a person speak, then translates that speech into printed language. The machine types what it hears someone say. Dyslexics of the 21st century will be able to speak and write without having to go through the actual process of writing. As new generations of voice writers are developed, dyslexics of the future will be able to dictate orally, and the machine will print out edited, corrected finished copy. No doubt hot debate will occur among adults who fear that such devices will only make students "lazy." The important issue is that language disabled students who have been chained by the enslaving disabilities of dyslexia will be set free to express themselves well in writing. Perhaps by the middle of the 21st century there will no longer be writing disability to crush the self-confidence of intelligent but handicapped writers.

Higher Education Opportunities for Dyslexics

In Chapter 7 we read fascinating stories about several dyslexics who overcame their disabilities. If Thomas A. Edison and George S.

Patton IV had been born in 1980, they would certainly have finished a college education. Beginning in the early 1980s several colleges and universities in the United States began to work with dyslexic students. A small Presbyterian school in Arkansas, The University of the Ozarks, has pioneered a special program for adult dyslexics. This has opened the door for similar programs in other schools. At The University of the Ozarks, Dr. Betty Robinson and her staff classify dyslexic students according to the level of disability. Severely dyslexic students are taught in a specially designed learning lab where all lectures are available on audiotape and full-time tutoring is available for each class. Each professor provides a written outline of each course, which allows dyslexics to see as well as hear important material several times. Tests and exams are administered orally with no time limit. Less severely disabled learners receive less help, and those with only moderate dyslexic problems receive help only as it is needed. Within this specially structured environment, several hundred dyslexic adults have been able to achieve a college degree.

It has required a great deal of work over a period of time, but those of us who believe in the worth of dyslexics have gradually convinced enough educators and administrators that this special population is worth the extra effort required to help them overcome their language disabilities. Today's elementary school and middle school students will find many opportunities for college study or vocational training. Following the model established by The University of the Ozarks, many colleges and universities began to provide special help for dyslexic students by the mid-1980s. For example, San Diego State University and the University of Arizona established excellent support programs for dyslexics. Numerous community colleges offer special help for learning disabled adults. As time goes by, more and more college-level programs for dyslexics will be established. Dyslexic students of the future will have no difficulty finding advanced educational opportunities. If Edison and Patton were children today, they would be actively recruited by colleges looking for gifted and talented dyslexic students. The 21st century will not waste priceless talent by failing to recognize dyslexic "diamonds in the rough," as our culture has done so often in the past.

The key to this new acceptance of dyslexia by adult education programs has been untimed exams and tests. By the early 1980s it was standard practice to offer untimed administration of such critical tests as the SAT and ACT, which colleges and universities use to screen applications for admission. Thousands of dyslexic students have significantly increased their SAT or ACT scores by taking the untimed form of those tests. It is not unusual to see a bright dyslexic 17-year-old almost double his or her ACT score with the untimed administration.

The field of professional admissions tests, such as LSAT for law school and MEDCAT for medical school, is also realizing the value of allowing untimed test administration for dyslexic applicants. Again, many highly intelligent dyslexics have demonstrated their potential for the study of law or medicine by increasing scores substantially when tests are untimed. State licensing exams are sometimes permitted to be untimed, although there is often reluctance on the part of governing boards to make this exception. I could tell remarkable stories of how dyslexic nurses, plumbers, real estate agents, accountants, and law students have earned their professional credentials through untimed proficiency tests. There was no way those bright adults could pass timed exams, but when the qualifying tests were given with no time limit, those highly skilled adults were able to demonstrate their knowledge. Dyslexics of the future will not have to face the arbitrary restrictions of being licensed or not on the basis of timed examinations.

Improved School Evaluation

With the implementation of Public Law 94-142 in the 1970s, public schools came under federal mandate to find and help all children with special problems. P.L. 94-142 clearly included dyslexia as a specific learning disability to be identified and remediated in "the least restrictive environment." For the first several years after this federal decree, most school districts in the United States were conscientious in trying to identify every child with special needs. A great deal of federal money was allocated to local school districts for this search. Each school established learning lab classrooms, now usually called resource rooms, where children with specific learning problems were taught separately. During the early 1980s the policies toward special education of learning disabled children began to shift away from separate classes toward mainstream teaching. The theory was that no child should be isolated from the mainstream of his or her peer group. Over a period of time, most self-contained classrooms for the special population were emptied back into the regular classrooms, and the wheel turned full circle. Teachers of my generation taught school with all students mixed together. Those with learning disabilities were mixed with those who had no learning problems. As we approach the 21st century, we are back to that teaching plan. Virtually every classroom teacher in the United States must deal with learning disabled students mixed with peers who have no learning problem. My generation had no training in how to deal with such a mixture. We just did the best we could, as I did the year I had 43 boys in one sixth-grade classroom. The best reader of that group scored middle third grade on the reading achievement test. Today many mainstream teachers face that kind of dilemma.

As this shift toward mainstream assignment has occurred, a rapid change has also occurred in the way students are evaluated for learning disability. Within the past decade a new profession has evolved, generally referred to as *school psychometry*. The school psychometrist is highly trained in administering certain kinds of diagnostic tests to screen large numbers of students for learning disability. As time goes by, the particular tests used will vary. The keystone test which supports the arch of school psychometry is the *Wechsler Intelligence Scale for Children* (WISC-R). Additional tests are also given to see how well the student performs with language skills, visual perception, auditory perception, and so forth. A typical psychometric evaluation might consist of the WISC-R, *Woodcock-Johnson Psycho-Educational Battery, Bender Gestalt Visual Motor Perceptual Test,* and the *Wide Range Achievement Test* (WRAT). Other tests may be added to this basic test group. This test administration produces several pages of statistics. Anyone who reviews these test findings must know how to interpret line after line and row after row of numbers and statistics. These tests survey certain skills and abilities quite well. In effect, each child's abilities are reduced to numbers. The child's performance is quantified and represented on paper by tightly packed numbers that are fed into a formula based upon a point system. If a child scores below a certain point level on this final scale, he or she is identified as having specific learning disability. If the child scores above the arbitrary cut-off point, then he or she is not identified as having learning disability. This mathematical process is highly efficient in scoring tests and translating test behavior into number equivalents. This system has proved excellent for purposes of assigning students to special programs, as well as administering large programs that must deal with hundreds of individuals.

The major flaw in the psychometric approach is that it leaves out several critical factors that must be considered when we determine learning disability in a child. In fact, the last place we should look for learning disability is at test scores themselves. Many professionals speak of "the kids who fall through the cracks." During the past 15 years, I have seen hundreds of severely learning disabled students who fell through the cracks of psychometric assessment. In my experience, the WISC-R fails to identify specific learning disability in 30% of the students screened by that test. This means that one-third of the truly dyslexic youngsters evaluated by the WISC-R do not show a typical learning disability pattern as the subtest profile is examined. Because so much faith is placed by most psychometrists in the WISC-R results, this approach often leaves out as many as one-third of the learning disabled population. When test scores are the major consideration for determining specific learning disability, this approach becomes clearly inadequate. A majority of the students who come to our diagnostic center have not been identified by the psychometric approach as having learning disability. Yet they cannot do acceptable classroom work. Their teachers are frustrated. These students cannot read, spell, write, copy, do math computation, listen well, or follow instructions adequately. Yet they score above the cut-off point on the psychometric scales used by various states to determine eligibility for special placement. Our clients in private practice are mostly those who fall through the cracks of standard psychometric evaluation (Hippchen, 1978; Jordan, 1974).

If test scores are the last place to look for learning disability, where should we begin our search? We should start at the most obvious point of all by watching the child do classroom tasks. Very few of the test activities of the standard psychometric evaluation format are the kinds of work the student is required to do several hours each day in the classroom. Learning disability is not a matter of intelligence or assembling puzzles or remembering how far it is from New York to London. Learning disability is being unable to read what the teacher assigns, control the pencil in writing, sound out words successfully, remember several things to do 10 minutes after the teacher gave the instructions, and so forth. Learning disability is seen in the level of restlessness that emerges as the day progresses. It is observed in the amount of daydreaming or "star gazing" the child does instead of staying on the task. Learning disability is a cluster of struggles. It includes many strands that must be seen to be identified. We cannot adequately infer learning disability by poring over sets of test scores and percentile rankings. We must discover whether a student is dyslexic by analyzing how classroom tasks are performed.

Psychometric evaluation has been honed into a precise system, and this new system has great value. However, the system now used by most schools to identify learning disability is incomplete. We need to add to it so that an overall picture of the child is obtained. Before it is determined whether or not a child has learning disability, the psychometrist must include behavioral descriptions from teachers who work with the child day after day. We must include guided observations from parents who live with the youngster the other 18 hours of every day. We must use observational instruments like the Slingerland Screening Tests (Slingerland, 1970) or the Jordan Written Screening Tests (Jordan, 1977, 1988b), which are designed to reveal specific dyslexic-like patterns. None of the tests now used by most psychometrists are designed to identify dyslexia. We also must include observational checklists that show Attention Deficit Disorder (Bloomingdale, 1984; Dykman, Ackerman, & Holcomb, 1985; Hagerman, 1983; Jordan, 1988a; Nickamin & James, 1984). We must have input from pediatricians and counselors who may have spotted such problems as Fragile X Syndrome or Tourette Syndrome (Hagerman, 1983). Our hope for the future is that the discipline of psychometry will continue to grow and mature. Psychometrists must take a new look at the many struggling, desperate youngsters who "fall through the cracks." These cracks must be sealed in the future to make sure that all children with special needs are adequately identified and treated (Boettcher, 1983; Oliphant, 1979; Rees, 1978).

References

Alston, J., & Taylor, J. (1987). *Handwriting: Theory, research and practice.* New York: Nichols.

American Psychiatric Association. (1980). *Diagnostic and statistical manual of mental disorders* (3rd ed.). Washington, DC: Author.

American Psychiatric Association. (1987). *Diagnostic and statistical manual of mental disorders* (3rd ed. rev.). Washington, DC: Author.

Blanchard, J.B., & Mannarino, F. (1978). Academic, perceptual, and visual levels of detained delinquents, In L.J. Hippchen (Ed.), *Ecological-biochemical approaches to treatment of delinquents and criminals* (pp. 341– 351). New York: Van Nostrand Reinhold.

Bloomingdale, L.M. (1984). *Attention deficit disorder.* Jamaica, NY: Spectrum.

Boettcher, J.V. (1983). Computer-based education: Classroom applications and benefits for the learning-disabled student. Proceedings of the 33rd annual conference of The Orton Dyslexia Society, *Annals of Dyslexia, 33,* 203–219.

Coppola, R. (1985). Recent developments in neuro-imaging techniques. In D.B. Gray & J.F. Kavanagh (Eds), *Biobehavioral measures of dyslexia* (pp. 63–69). Parkton, MD: York.

Cott, A. (1978). Symptoms and treatment of children with learning disorders. In L.S. Hippchen (Ed.), *Ecological-biochemical approaches to treatment of delinquents and criminals* (pp. 61–74). New York: Van Nostrand Reinhold.

Critchley, M. (1970). *The dyslexic child.* London: Heinemann.

Denckla, M.B. (1985). Issues of overlap and heterogeneity in dyslexia. In D.B. Gray & J.F. Kavanagh (Eds.), *Biobehavioral measures of dyslexia* (pp. 41–46). Parkton, MD: York.

Duane, D.D. (1979). Toward a definition of dyslexia: A summary of views. In A. Ansara (Ed.), *Bulletin of The Orton Dyslexia Society* (pp. 56–64). Baltimore, MD: Author.

Duane, D.D. (1985, November). *Psychiatric implications of neurological difficulties.* Symposium conducted at The Menninger Foundation, Topeka, KS.

Duane, D.D. (1987, November). *The anatomy of dyslexia and neurobiology of human aptitude.* Symposium conducted by The Orton Dyslexia Society, San Francisco.

Duane, D.D., & Rome, P.D. (1985). *The dyslexic child.* Cambridge, MA: Educators Publishing Service.

Dykman, R., Ackerman, P.T., & Holcomb, P.J. (1985). Reading disabled and ADD children: Similarities and differences. In D.B. Gray & J.F. Kavanagh (Eds.), *Biobehavioral measures of dyslexia* (pp. 47–62). Parkton, MD: York.

Enfield, M.L. (1987, November). *The quest for literacy.* Symposium conducted by The Orton Dyslexia Society, San Francisco.

Evans, M.M. (1982). *Dyslexia: An annotated bibliography.* Westport, CT: Greenwood.

Galaburda, A. (1983). Developmental dyslexia: Current anatomical research. Proceedings of the 33rd annual conference of The Orton Dyslexia Society, *Annals of Dyslexia, 33,* 41–54.

Geiger, G., & Lettvin, J.Y. (1987). Peripheral vision in persons with dyslexia. *The New England Journal of Medicine, 316* (20), 1238–1243.

Geschwind, N. (1979). Asymmetries of the brain: New developments. In A. Ansara (Ed.), *Bulletin of The Orton Dyslexia Society* (pp. 67–73). Baltimore, MD: The Orton Dyslexia Society.

Geschwind, N. (1983). Biological associations of left-handedness. Proceedings of the 33rd annual conference of The Orton Dyslexia Society, *Annals of Dyslexia, 33,* 29–40.

Geschwind, N. (1984). *Why Orton was right.* Baltimore, MD: The Orton Dyslexia Society.

Geschwind, N. (1985). The biology of dyslexia: The unfinished manuscript. In D.B. Gray & J.F. Kavanagh (Eds.), *Biobehavioral measures of dyslexia* (pp. 21–24). Parkton, MD: York.

Gray, D.B., & Kavanagh, J.F. (Eds.), *Biobehavioral measures of dyslexia.* Parkton, MD: York.

Greenstein, T.N. (1976). *Vision and learning disability.* St. Louis: American Optometric Association.

Grimm, V.E. (1986, March). *Behavioral toxicology: Relevance to learning disabilities.* Symposium conducted by the Association for Children and Adults with Learning Disabilities, New York.

Hagerman, R.J. (1983, March). *Developmental pediatrics.* A symposium conducted by New Frontiers, Steamboat Springs, CO.

Harris, T. L., & Hodges, R. E. (Eds.). (1981). *A dictionary of reading and related terms.* Newark, NJ: International Reading Association.

Hippchen, L. J. (1978). A model for community programs dealing with antisocial persons. In L. J. Hippchen (Ed.), *Ecological-biochemical approaches to treatment of delinquents and criminals* (pp. 371–388). New York: Van Nostrand Reinhold.

Hynd, G., & Cohen, M. (1983). *Dyslexia: Neuropsychological theory, research, and clinical differentiation.* New York: Grune & Stratton.

Inhelder, B., & Piaget, J. (1974). *The early growth of logic in the child* (pp. 102–114). New York: Harper & Row.

Inouye, D. K., & Sorenson, M. R. (1985). Profiles of dyslexia: The computer as an instrument of vision. In D. B. Gray & J. F. Kavanagh (Eds.), *Biobehavioral measures of dyslexia* (pp. 297–322). Parkton, MD: York.

Jansky, J. J. (1988). Overview of early prediction and intervention. In R. L. Masland & M. W. Masland (Eds.), *Prevention of reading failure* (pp. 219–224). Parkton, MD: York.

Jernigan, S. (1985, November). *Measures of brain function: Understanding the influence of brain dysfunction on behavior and learning problems.* Symposium conducted by The Menninger Foundation, Topeka, KS.

Johnson, I. T., & Stetson, E. G. (1984). *Type-write program.* Austin, TX: PRO-ED.

Jordan, D. R. (1974). *Learning disabilities and predelinquent behavior of juveniles.* Oklahoma City, OK: Oklahoma Association for Children with Learning Disabilities.

Jordan, D. R. (1977). *Dyslexia in the classroom* (2nd ed.). Columbus, OH: Merrill.

Jordan, D. R. (1988a). *Attention deficit disorder.* Austin, TX: PRO-ED.

Jordan, D. R. (1988b). *Jordan prescriptive/tutorial reading program for moderate and severe dyslexics.* Austin, TX: PRO-ED.

Keogh, B. K., Sears, S., & Royal, N. (1987). Slingerland screening and instructional approaches for children at-risk for school. In R. L. Masland & M. W. Masland (Eds.), *Prevention of reading failure* (pp. 107–120). Parkton, MD: York.

Kutchins, H., & Kirk, S. (1988). The future of DSM: Scientific and professional issues. *The Harvard Medical School Mental Health Letter* (p. 3).

Leisman, G. (1976). *Basic visual processes and learning disability.* Springfield, IL: Thomas.

Lundberg, I. (1988). Preschool prevention of reading failure: Does training in phonological awareness work? In R. L. Masland & M. W. Masland (Eds.), *Prevention of reading failure* (pp. 163–174). Parkton, MD: York.

Masland, R. L., & Masland, M. W. (Eds.). (1988). *Prevention of reading failure.* Parkton, MD: York.

McEwen, B. S. (1986, March). *Neuroendocrinology.* Symposium conducted by the Association for Children and Adults with Learning Disability, New York.

Missildine, W. H., & Galton, L. (1972). *Your inner child of the past.* New York: Simon & Schuster.

Nichamin, S.J., & Windell, J. (1984). *A new look at attention deficit disorder.* Waterford, ME: Minerva.

Ochroch, R. (1981). *The diagnosis and treatment of minimal brain dysfunction in children.* New York: Human Sciences Press.

Oliphant, G.G. (1979). Program planning for dyslexic children in the general classroom. In A. Ansara (Ed.), *Bulletin of The Orton Dyslexia Society* (pp. 225– 237). Baltimore, MD: The Orton Dyslexia Society.

Orton Dyslexia Society. (1988). *Winter newsletter.* Baltimore, MD: Author.

Osman, B. (1986). Learning disabilities in adolescents generate socialization disorders. *Hill Top Spectrum, 4* (2), 3.

Philpott, W.H. (1978). Ecological aspects of antisocial behavior. In L.J. Hippchen (Ed.), *Ecological-biochemical approaches to treatment of delinquents and criminals* (pp. 116–137). New York: Van Nostrand Reinhold.

Rayner, K. (1983). Eye movements, perceptual span, and reading disability. Proceedings of the 33rd annual conference of The Orton Dyslexia Society. *Annals of Dyslexia, 33,* 163–174.

Rees, E.L. (1978). Early diagnosis and treatment of childhood disorders. In A. Ansara (Ed.), *Bulletin of The Orton Society* (pp. 43–50). Baltimore, MD: The Orton Dyslexia Society.

Shucard, D.W., Cummins, K.R., Gay, E., Lairsmith, J., & Welanko, P. (1985). Electro-physiological studies of reading disabled children: In search of subtypes. In D.B. Gray & J.F. Kavanagh (Eds.), *Biobehavioral measures of dyslexia* (pp. 86–106). Parkton, MD: York.

Silver, L. (1985, March). *The learning disabled adult: Who is he? What is he?* Symposium conducted by The Menninger Foundation, Topeka, KS.

Slavin, S.H. (1978). Information processing defects in delinquents. In L.J. Hippchen (Ed.), *Ecological-biochemical approaches to treatment of delinquents and criminals* (pp. 75–104). New York: Van Nostrand Reinhold.

Slingerland, B.H. (1970). *Slingerland screening tests for identifying children with specific language disability.* Cambridge, MA: Educators Publishing Service.

Steeves, J. (1987, November). *Computers: Powerful tools for dyslexic children.* Symposium conducted by The Orton Dyslexia Society, San Francisco.

Thurber, D.N. (1984). *D'Nealian manuscript: A continuous stroke approach to handwriting.* Novato, CA: Academic Therapy Publications.

Wacker, J. (1975). *The dyslogic syndrome.* Texas Association for Children with Learning Disabilities. Dallas, TX: Author.

Wilson, B.C., & Risucci, D.A. (1988). The early identification of developmental language disorders and the prediction of the acquisition of reading skills. In R.L. Masland & M.W. Masland (Eds.), *Prevention of reading failure* (pp. 187–203). Parkton, MD: York.

Wunderlich, R.C. (1978). Neuroallergy as a contributing factor to social misfits: Diagnosis and treatment. In L.J. Hippchen (Ed.), *Ecological-biochemical approaches to treatment of delinquents and criminals* (pp. 229–253). New York: Van Nostrand Reinhold.

APPENDIX 1
Checklist of Visual Dyslexia Symptoms

The following informal checklist can help parents and teachers identify visual dyslexia. It is important to withhold judgment until a definite syndrome of dyslexic symptoms has been identified in a student's behavior. If a significant cluster of perceptual errors appears as the adult studies a student's performance, then it is generally safe to conclude that visual dyslexia exists.

____ **Confusion with Sequence**

- ____ has poor concept of time
- ____ has poor concept of chronological order of events
- ____ cannot give day, month, and year of birth
- ____ cannot write months of year
- ____ cannot write days of week
- ____ cannot remember multiplication tables

____ **Difficulty Following Directions** (This can also indicate Attention Deficit Disorder—ADD Syndrome.)

- ____ cannot remember daily routines at home
- ____ cannot follow teacher's directions in classroom
- ____ cannot comprehend instructions when given to a group; must have one-to-one explanations
- ____ needs constant reminding of what to do

____ **Faulty Oral Language**

- ____ loses words, "goes blank," while telling, naming, describing
- ____ can tell stories or give oral reports, but gets details in wrong sequence
- ____ has difficulty with correct sequence of events

_____ **Faulty Reading Comprehension**

_____ fails to identify main ideas

_____ tells story details out of sequence

_____ loses meaning of sentences or paragraphs before reaching the end

_____ fails to draw inferences from what has been read

_____ has difficulty recalling details when answering comprehension questions

_____ **Slow Work Rate**

_____ seldom finishes timed exercises

_____ easily frustrated when pressured for speed

_____ work pace considerably slower than classmates

_____ can do satisfactory work if given ample time and help

_____ will not use full time allowance on timed tests; guesses, marking items at random

_____ **Difficulty with Alphabet**

_____ does not know alphabet in correct sequence

_____ omits certain letters from alphabetic sequence

_____ mixes capital and lowercase letters

_____ mixes manuscript and cursive styles

_____ confuses similar letters

_____ writes certain letters backwards or upside down

_____ sings alphabet song or repeats rhyme to check sequence

_____ is not able to synchronize voice, finger, and eyes while checking work

____ **Confusion with Symbols**

- ____ demonstrates poor perception when symbols are traced on back
  - ____ mental image is upside down
  - ____ mental image is backwards
  - ____ distorts shapes of symbols
  - ____ turns symbols over
- ____ writes capital *B* and *D* instead of lowercase *b* and *d*
- ____ confuses symbols in reading, writing, and arithmetic
- ____ cannot conserve the form in copy work (loses mental images as eyes refocus)
- ____ confuses similar symbols
  - ____ *b–d–p–q*
  - ____ *h–y*
  - ____ *r–n*
  - ____ *r–c–s*
  - ____ *f–t*
  - ____ *3–E*
  - ____ *h–n*
  - ____ *m–w*
  - ____ *l–i*
  - ____ *n–u*
  - ____ *N–Z*
  - ____ *6–9*
  - ____ +, ×, ÷

____ **Errors in Oral Reading**

- ____ reverses whole words
- ____ reverses beginning letters
- ____ transposes *l* and *r* in consonant blends
- ____ substitutes similar letters or words
- ____ transposes letters inside words
- ____ fails to see small details in words
- ____ fails to see punctuation marks
- ____ omits endings
- ____ telescopes (leaves out letters or syllables)
- ____ perseverates (adds extra letters or syllables)

____ **Errors in Spelling**

- ____ transposes silent letters within words
- ____ does not recall correct order of letters
- ____ misplaces silent *e*

____ **Errors in Arithmetic**

- ____ reverses the process while working problems
- ____ carries or borrows wrong digit
- ____ cannot organize facts in story problems
- ____ misreads signs (plus for ×, times for +, subtract for +)

____ **Errors in Copying**

- ____ loses place on board (far point)
- ____ misspells on paper
- ____ fails to observe capital letters
- ____ fails to observe punctuation marks
- ____ fails to space properly
- ____ erases frequently
- ____ overprints to correct mistakes
- ____ reverses letters
- ____ reverses whole words
- ____ telescopes
- ____ perseverates
- ____ works unusually slowly
- ____ tries to avoid copying tasks

APPENDIX 2
Checklist of Auditory Dyslexia Symptoms

The following checklist can help parents and teachers identify patterns associated with auditory dyslexia. It is important to withhold judgment until a definite syndrome of symptoms has been identified.

____ **Confusion with Phonics**

- ____ cannot distinguish differences in vowel sounds
    - ____ does not hear long vowel sounds
    - ____ does not hear short vowel sounds
    - ____ does not hear schwa vowel sounds
    - ____ does not hear changes in vowel sounds
- ____ cannot distinguish differences in consonant sounds
- ____ does not hear differences between similar consonant sounds:
    - ____ /b/ /d/
    - ____ /b/ /p/
    - ____ /d/ /t/
    - ____ /g/ /k/
    - ____ /m/ /n/
    - ____ /f/ /v/
    - ____ /s/ /z/
    - ____ /th/ /f/
- ____ does not hear the sounds within consonant clusters
- ____ cannot interpret diacritical markings
- ____ cannot interpret phonetic respellings

____ **Confusion with Words**

- ____ cannot tell when words are alike or different
- ____ cannot hear or say rhyming words
- ____ gives garbled pronunciation (echolalia)

____ **Confusion with Spelling**

- ____ writes very slowly
- ____ depends upon memory tricks to recall spellings

_____ cannot apply phonics rules when spelling

_____ tends to spell phonetically

_____ breaks consonant clusters when spelling (transposes *l* and *r*—*paly* for *play, bran* for *barn, gril* for *girl*)

_____ confuses sounds of consonant letters:

_____ *c* for *k* _____ *f* for *v*

_____ *m* for *n* _____ *d* for *t*

_____ *s* for *z* _____ *f* for *th*

_____ does not hear sounds of /m/, /n/, /l/, /w/, or /r/

_____ leaves out sounds when writing words (telescopes)

_____ adds sounds when writing words (perseverates)

_____ does not hear accent in words

_____ does not hear vowel sounds within words

_____ does not hear syllables within words

_____ does not remember different or unusual spellings

_____ cannot retain memory of basic spelling words

_____ asks speaker to repeat

_____ erases, marks over, crosses out

_____ tries to hide work while writing

_____ **Reinforcement While Writing or Reading**

_____ whispers while reading silently

_____ whispers while writing

APPENDIX 3
Checklist of Dysgraphia Characteristics

This checklist can help parents and teachers identify dysgraphia.

_____ **Difficulty with Alphabet or Number Symbols**

- _____ does not remember how to write certain letters or numerals
- _____ distorts shapes of certain letters or numerals
- _____ overall writing is awkward, uneven
- _____ has difficulty transferring from manuscript to cursive style
- _____ continues to print manuscript style long after introduction to cursive style
- _____ certain letters or numerals are fragmented
- _____ writing resembles "bird scratching"; is virtually illegible
- _____ has difficulty distinguishing between capital and lowercase letters
- _____ mixes capital and lowercase letters

_____ **Confusion with Directionality**

- _____ writes certain letters, numerals, or words backwards (mirror image)
- _____ tends to write on mirror side (left side) of vertical midline when moving to next column
- _____ marks from bottom to top when forming certain letters or numerals
- _____ uses backwards (clockwise) motions when writing circular strokes in certain letters or numerals
- _____ continually erases or overprints to change what was written first
- _____ writing slants up, down, or wobbles up and down

____ **Sentence Structure**

- ____ composes meaningful content in spite of poor handwriting
- ____ transposes grammatical elements within sentences, but produces good overall meaning
- ____ tends to use complete sentences instead of fragments

____ **Difficulty Conserving Form in Copying Simple Shapes**

- ____ distorts simple shapes
- ____ fails to close corners
- ____ draws "ears" where lines meet or change direction
- ____ has difficulty reproducing simple designs from memory
- ____ work deteriorates toward end of writing exercise
- ____ has difficulty staying on lines when tracing

____ **Tendency to Telescope**

- ____ omits letters when writing words
- ____ omits syllables or sound units when writing words
- ____ runs letters and words together
- ____ runs words together (usually when copying)

____ **Tendency to Perseverate**

- ____ adds unnecessary letters or sound units to written words
- ____ repeats the same letters or syllables in written words
- ____ adds unnecessary sound units to spoken words
- ____ repeats syllables or sound units in spoken words
- ____ falls into parrotlike repetition of rhyming sounds during games or conversation

Author Index

Subject Index